A Colo
Meat Ii

J Infante Gil
Principal Veterinarian of
Meat Inspection of
the Lisbon Council

J Costa Durão
Head Professor of
Morbid Anatomy
Lisbon Veterinary School

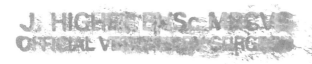

M WOLFE

Copyright © J. Infante Gil, J. Costa Durão, 1990
Published by Wolfe Publishing, Ltd 1990
First published in Portuguese (© 1985) as
'Manual de Inspecção Sanitária de Carnes' by
Fundação Calouste Gulbenkian, Lisbon, Portugal
Printed by Grafos, Arte Sobre Papel, Barcelona, Spain
Reprinted 1994 by Mosby–Year Book Europe Ltd.
ISBN 0 7234 1525 0

A CIP catalogue record for this book is available
from the British Library.

For a full list of Atlases, plus forthcoming titles,
please write to: Mosby–Year Book Europe Ltd,
Lynton House, 7-12 Tavistock Square, London WC1H 9LB,
England.

CONTENTS

PREFACE

This book is primarily intended for those studying or working in meat inspection, but will also prove valuable to anyone involved with animal pathology. The pictures have been collected over a period of more than 20 years, and cover most pathological conditions likely to occur in day-to-day meat inspection, both before and after slaughter. A few pictures of cases involving natural death are included.

The captions identify the species, the body parts or viscera shown and the diagnosis of the pathology involved. A concise description of the relevant pathological changes found is included. When they are relevant, alternative pathologies have been listed in order to assist the meat inspector in making a differential diagnosis.

The 'decisions' referred to in the captions are based on the recommendations included in the 'International code of practice for ante-mortem and post-mortem judgement of slaughter animals and meat', which were adopted during my own professional activity as a meat inspector. These decisions should not be regarded as absolute certainties but as general guidelines for the meat inspector. In the text, the decision always relates to the whole animal or its carcase, including its head and viscera, and not only the parts shown in the photograph.

The decision is omitted in cases where insufficient information was available.

J. Infante Gil
Lisbon, 1989

INTRODUCTION

The inspection of animals destined for slaughter, their carcases and offal must be systematic to ensure that products intended for human consumption are safe. It should also protect the processing industry from economic loss due to the supply of inferior meat products.

Systematic inspection should include measures to protect food handlers, especially slaughterhouse workers, from occupational infections. Consideration must also be given to the containment of infections, and the recognition of hereditary disease and poisoning among livestock. Inspection, both ante-mortem and post-mortem can provide important information for the animal breeder, such as the lean-to-fat and lean-to-bone ratios and the general quality of the meat. Quality is, of course, necessary in order to maintain product standards, and meet the consumers' demands (colour, texture, moisture content, smell, tenderness, etc.). Equally important is the collection of data on the chemical constituents of the meat, such as the relative proportion of proteins, lipids, minerals and vitamins.

The relative proportions of lean to fat and bone are especially useful in the detection of pathological changes.

The species generally considered for slaughter are bovine, porcine, ovine, caprine and equine. Some countries also include animals such as reindeer, camel, buffalo, moose, deer, bear, etc. There are also numerous religious constraints on the consumption of meat.

In order to establish a uniform set of criteria, the following terms and expressions have been adopted throughout this book:

1 *Abattoir*: premises approved and registered by the controlling authority used for the slaughter of animals for human consumption.

2 *Brand*: any mark or stamp approved by the controlling authority (includes any tag or label bearing such a mark or stamp).

3 *Carcase*: the body of any slaughtered animal after bleeding and dressing.

4 *Cleaning*: the removal of objectionable matter.

5 *Condemned*: a slaughter animal or meat that has been inspected and judged as unfit for human consumption and branded accordingly. (*Total condemnation* involves the entire carcase and offal; *partial condemnation* involves only specified parts.)

6 *Contamination*: the direct or indirect transmission of objectionable matter.

7 *Controlling authority*: the official authority charged by the Government with the control of hygiene, including meat inspection, within the abattoir or establishment.

8 *Detained*: under the control and security of the controlling authority pending final judgement.

9 *Disinfection*: the reduction, without adversely affecting the food, by means of hygienically satisfactory chemical agents and/or physical methods, of the number of microorganisms to a level that will not lead to harmful contamination of food.

10 *Dressed* or *dressing*
(a) in relation to slaughtered animals – except for pigs, sheep and lambs, goats and kids – dressing means the removal of the head, hide or skin, viscera (with or without kidneys), genital organs, urinary bladder and feet up to the carpal and tarsal joints, and udders of lactating animals, animals which have given birth or are in advanced pregnancy.
(b) in relation to slaughtered pigs, dressing means the removal of hair and bristles or skin, claws, eyelids, viscera (with or without kidneys), genital organs, urinary bladder, udders in the case of lactating animals, animals that have farrowed or are in advanced pregnancy, and the external acoustic duct unless an alternative effective form of cleaning it is carried out.
(c) in relation to sheep and lambs, goats and kids dressing means the removal of the head (except in the case of young lambs and young kids), the pelt or skin, including that of the head, viscera (with or without the kidneys), genital organs, urinary bladder and feet up to the carpal and tarsal joints, and udders of lactating animals, animals that have given birth or are in advanced pregnancy.
(d) in relation to cattle, pigs and solipeds dressing includes, where necessary, splitting of the carcase. To split means to divide the carcase lengthwise in the medial line.

11 *Edible offal*: such offal as has been passed as fit for human consumption.

12 *Establishment*: any premises approved and registered by the controlling authority for the preparation, handling, packing or storage of fresh meat.

13 *Fresh meat*: meat which has not been treated for the purposes of preservation. Meat which has been refrigerated should still be regarded as fresh for the purposes of this definition.

14 *Inspector*: a properly trained officer appointed by the controlling authority of a country for the purposes of meat inspection and hygiene control. The supervision of meat hygiene including the inspection of meat should be the responsibility of an official veterinarian.

15 *Manager*: any person currently responsible for the running of the abattoir or establishment.

16 *Meat*: the edible part of any mammal slaughtered in an abattoir.

17 *Offal*: any edible or non-edible part of the animal other than the carcase.

18 *Potable water*: water that is pure and wholesome at the point of use in accordance with WHO requirements for drinking water.

19 *Protective clothing*: special garments, including head coverings and footwear, used as outer wear by persons in an abattoir or establishment and intended to prevent the contamination of meat.

20 *Residues*: any foreign substance (including its metabolites), therapeutic or prophylactic agents which are objectionable or a hazard to human health, remaining in slaughter animals prior to slaughter, either as a result of treatment or accidental exposure. Examples of such substances are: antibiotics, anthelmintics, growth promoters, hormones, hormone-like substances, pesticides, tranquillizers, radioactive materials, chemotherapeutics, tenderizers and disinfectants.

21 *Slaughter*: killing of a slaughter animal for the purposes of human consumption (includes bleeding).

22 *Slaughter animal*: any mammal brought into an abattoir for slaughter.

23 *Viscera*: the organs of the thoracic and abdominal cavities.

ACKNOWLEDGEMENTS

We wish to thank Professors A Martins Mendes and M C Peleteiro for their contributions to this book.

Many thanks are also due to the National Laboratory of Veterinary Research and the Laboratory of Morbid Anatomy of the Veterinary School, Lisbon, for the histological work which they undertook specifically for us.

The style of the book precludes an extensive bibliography, but we must acknowledge the following invaluable sources:

1 International code of practice for ante-mortem and post-mortem judgement of slaughter-animals and meat

2 Code d'usages internationaux récommandes en matière d'hygiene pour la viande fraiche, l'inspection ante-mortem des animaux d'abattoir et les produits carnes traités.

3 CAC/RCP11/13

4 Commission du codex alimentarius

1: Ante-mortem inspection

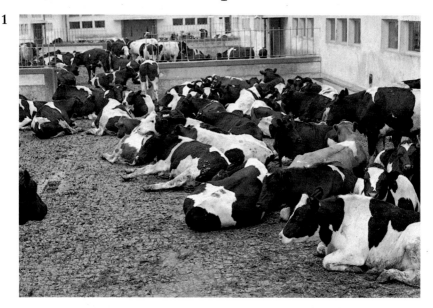

1 Exhaustion: cattle A consignment of cattle recently unloaded after a long trip by sea. Their drowsiness and almost permanently supine position led to a suspicion of exhaustion which was confirmed by tests performed on the meat from two bullocks (final pH and boiling test).

Decision: Authorization for slaughter was delayed for 3 days for resting purposes. The animals fasted the day before slaughter and there was a fresh ante-mortem inspection.

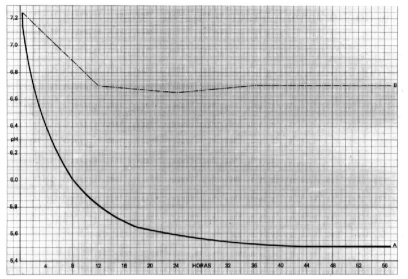

2 The 'A' curve represents the normal post-mortem pH decline, determined in samples of the longissimus dorsi muscle at the level of the 12th intercostal space from carcases of adult bovines (slaughtered in healthy condition), which were refrigerated in a cold chamber at 1°C. and 90% relative humidity. Under such circumstances, the final pH is achieved around 44 hours post-slaughter. The final pH does not change appreciably for several years in frozen carcases kept at temperatures below −18°C.

The 'B' curve represents the post-mortem pH decline following the same procedures, in a wild bull which had been submitted to intense physical exertion (bullfight) 10 hours before slaughter. This indicates an insufficiency of muscular glycogen and/or partial inactivation of glycolitic enzymes.

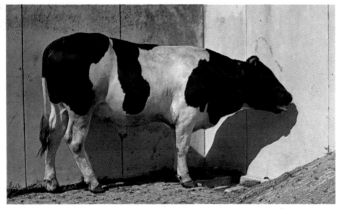

3 Dyspnoea due to effort: ox   The animal assumed an orthopnoeic attitude, with considerable respiration increase.

Decision: Authorization for slaughter was delayed to assess the influence of adequate rest.

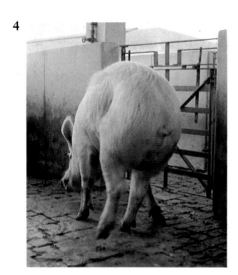

4 Ataxia: boar   The animal showed a difficult and arrhythmic walk, and uncoordinated movement.

Hypothetical diagnosis: traumatic changes affecting the muscles and ligaments of the pelvic girdle (confirmed in the post-mortem inspection). Neural disturbances. Traumatization of the skull.

Decision: Slaughter was authorized with special precautions.

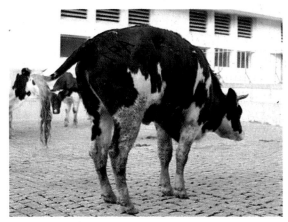

5 **Ischuria: cow** Animal in permanent urinating position, making unsuccessful efforts to pass urine.

Differential diagnosis: Rabies; Abscess in the spinal cord; Labour; Defaecation; Colic.

Decision: Condemnation at ante-mortem inspection. A delay in the slaughter authorization may be considered.

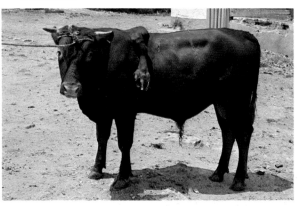

6 **Supranumerary limb (polymelia) – withers: ox** An extra anterior limb can be seen attached to the withers, in the left costal region.

Decision: Slaughter authorized with special precautions, considering the abnormality.

7

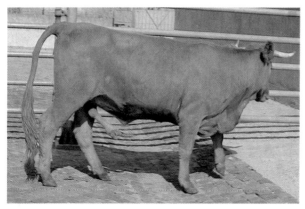

7 Supranumerary limb (polymelia) – pelvis (pelvic girdle): cattle Attached through a pseudojoint to the pelvis. An extra limb of reduced dimensions can be seen.

Decision: Slaughter authorized under special precautions, considering the abnormality.

8

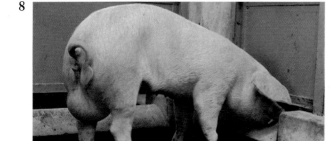

8 Ventral hernia: swine A voluminous swelling in the posterior abdominal wall ends slightly under the vulva. The detailed examination eliminated a diagnosis of hermaphroditism, because the contents of the hernial sac were reduced by compression and borborygmi were heard during auscultation. A ventral hernia was located under the skin caused by the passage of a segment of the gut through the abdominal wall.

Differential diagnosis: Neoplasia; Abscess; Orchitis.

Decision: Slaughter authorized under special precautions, considering the swelling.

9 Emaciation: cow Animal had reduced liveliness, slow movements, was extremely lean, without palpable accumulations of subcutaneous fat. The spinous processes of the lumbar vertebrae can be clearly seen through the skin and the hair was thick but lacking lustre. A mucopurulent liquid dripped from the mouth.

Decision: Condemnation or, alternatively, authorization for slaughter delayed.

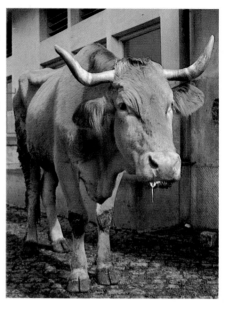

9

10 Intoxication: cattle The animal is defaecating, and large amounts of seromucous liquid are being expelled. She also displays sialorrhoea in a typical situation of accidental intoxication with organophosphates.

Differential diagnosis: Rift Valley fever; Anaphylactic reaction; Foot and mouth disease; Stomatitis.

Decision: Authorization for slaughter delayed.

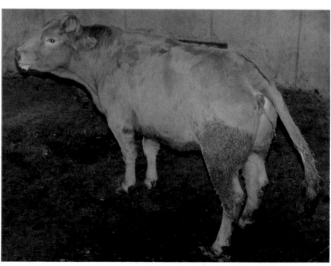

10

11

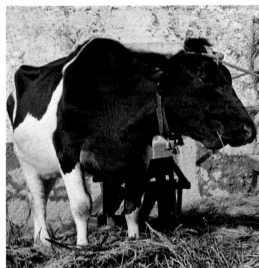

11 Traumatic pericarditis: cow The animal was depressed and apathetic, with dyspnoea and oedema at the entry of the thorax and in the subglossal region. The jugular veins were enlarged (stasis), the cardiac percussion area enlarged and the cardiac sounds indistinct. Rectal temperature was normal.

Decision: Condemnation.

12

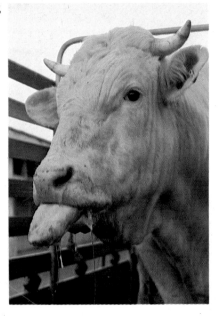

12 Foot and mouth disease (aphthous fever): ox This animal was condemned at the ante-mortem inspection because of hyperthermia, sialorrhoea (viscous saliva) and persistent protrusion of the tongue. The laboratory confirmed the diagnosis of foot and mouth disease through the identification of the virus. In the hypothetical diagnosis other possibilities were considered such as: actinobacillosis, non-specific glossitis and intoxication by organophosphates, etc.

13 Aphthous glossitis: ox Tongue of the ox shown in the previous picture. When the tongue was removed from the oral cavity, areas of the mucosa sloughed off. The enlargement and congestion of the organ were very marked. G and P : lymph nodes.

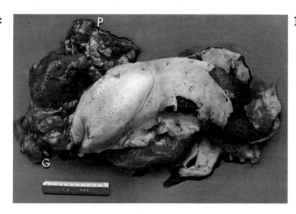

14 Aphthous fever – sialorrhoea: cattle Apart from sialorrhoea the animal was feverish, with gingivitis and ulceronecrotic glossitis.

Differential diagnosis: Peripharyngeal–laryngeal oedema; Unspecific stomatitis; Rinderpest; Mucosal disease.

Decision: Condemnation in the ante-mortem inspection.

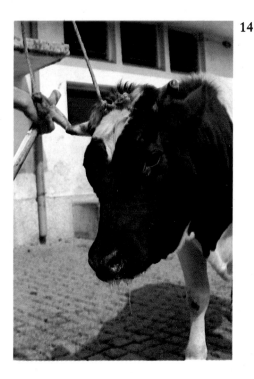

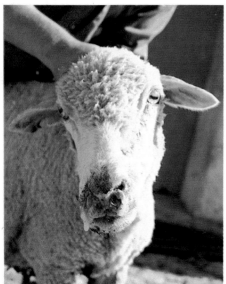

15 Rhinorrhoea – nostrils: sheep The animal presented a bilateral discharge of serous nasal mucus, which usually occurs in severe cases of lungworm infection.

Decision: Slaughter authorized under special precautions.

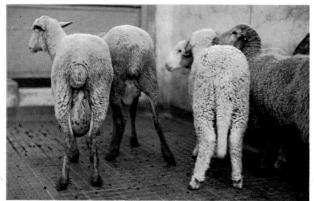

16 Mastitis – udder: ewe The ewe on the left was affected by an acute inflammatory disease of the mammary gland, which was markedly enlarged with congestion of the udder. The ewe on its right had chronic mastitis of the right udder, which was atrophic and firm despite the suppurative mastitis that was, meanwhile, affecting the left udder.

Decision: Condemnation.

17 Septic mastitis – udder: ewe The mammary gland belonging to the ewe shown on the left of the previous picture was affected by a developing mastitis, with abscesses and marked sclerosis, characteristic of mastitis by *Corynebacterium ovis*.

Decision: Condemnation. (Animals slaughtered in sanitary abattoir.)

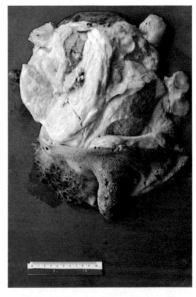

18 Mastitis – udder: ewe The left udder of the ewe shown on the right of **16** was affected by a purulent focal infection, accompanied by proliferating reaction of the fibrous connective tissue. The nodular profile of the right udder and its obvious atrophy are characteristic of a chronic catarrhal mastitis.

Decision: Condemnation.

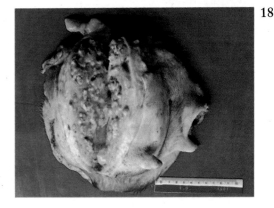

19

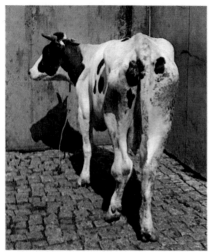

19 Arthritis – hock joint:
cow The animal avoided standing on the left pelvic limb due to an inflammatory reaction of the hock joint. The muscles of the affected limb were considerably atrophic, in contrast to the right one.

Differential diagnosis: Arthrosis; Neoplasia.

Decision: Slaughter authorized under special precautions.

20

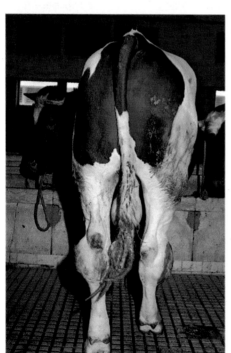

20 Polyarthritis – hock joints:
ox The animal showed considerable swelling of both hock joints which presented clear fluctuation.

Differential diagnosis: Arthrosis; Neoplasias.

Decision: Authorization for slaughter delayed.

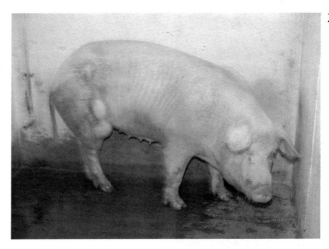

21 Swellings and arthritis – flank and joints: swine The animal presented with localized swellings and fluctuation in the stifle joint and knee on the right side and also marked hypertrophy of the prefemoral lymph node. A few abscesses were also noticed in the flank.

Decision: Condemnation.

22 Enlargement of the scrotum: swine The left scrotal pouch was considerably enlarged compared to the right one.

Hypothetical diagnosis: Orchitis; hydrocele; Spermatocele: hernia; neoplasia; cyst.

Decision: Slaughter authorized with special precautions.

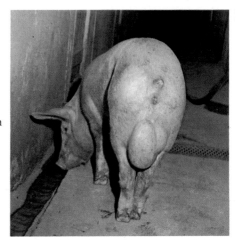

23

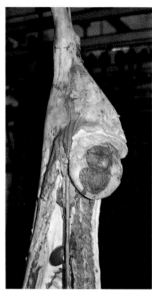

23 Necrotic orchitis – testicles: swine The left testicle of the animal shown in the previous figure was affected by a necrotic inflammatory reaction and surrounded by marked fibrosis.

Decision: Approval with elimination of the affected tissues (post-mortem).

24 Neoformation – intermandibular region: cow A highly exophitic mushroom-like tumour covered by a thick skin, was attached to the submandibular region of this cow.

Hypothetical diagnosis: Actinobacillosis or actinomycosis; keloid; abscess; neoplasia.

Decision: Slaughter authorized with special precautions.

24

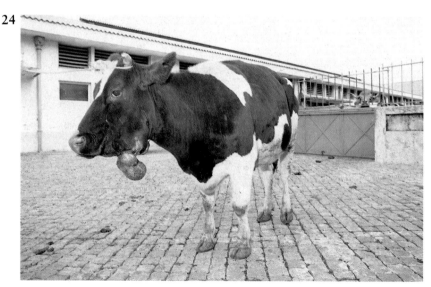

25 Actinobacillosis – neoformation: cow The cut surface of the tumour shown in the previous picture disclosed a pale, hard, compact tissue where greyish-red nodules were disseminated.

Differential diagnosis: Neoplasia; keloid.

Decision: Approval (in the post-mortem inspection) with elimination of the head (including tongue).

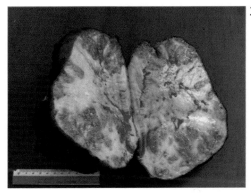

26 Dermatophytosis (ringworm) – skin: cattle The lesions presented by the animal, which was clearly underfed, were extensive areas of alopecia and thickened skin. The diagnosis of ringworm was confirmed through identification of *Tricophyton verrucosum*.

Differential diagnosis: Dermatitis.

Decision: Slaughter authorized with special precautions.

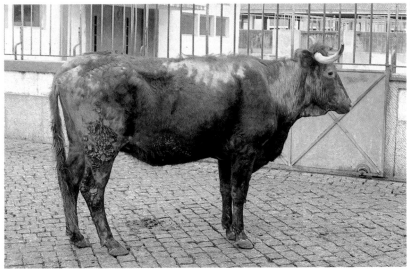

27

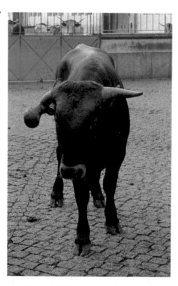

27 Neoformation – horn: ox In the short and thickened right horn, a corneal growth could be seen close to the extremity, ending in a spherical horny tumour.

Decision: Slaughter authorized with special precautions.

28

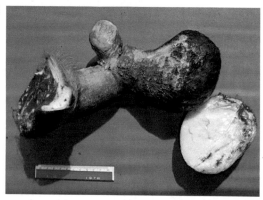

28 Hard fibroma: ox Section of the neoplasia shown in the previous picture, fibrous and hard, with white and dry surface. A benign neoplasia was confirmed by histopathological examination.

Differential diagnosis: Osteosarcoma.

Decision: Approval with elimination of the affected horn (post-mortem).

29 Tumefaction – upper jaw: sheep The tumefaction located in the right cheek showed well-defined and regular limits, a hard consistency and was attached to the upper jaw.

Hypothetical diagnosis: Neoplasia; Keloid; Abscess.

Decision: Slaughter authorized with special precautions.

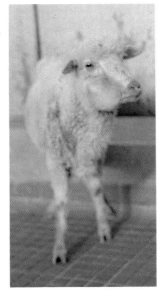

30 Osteoma – upper jaw: sheep After slaughter, an incision in the tumefaction (**29**) showed hard tissue, yellow-pink, arising from the upper jaw.

Differential diagnosis: Malignant neoplasia.

Decision: Approval with elimination of the head.

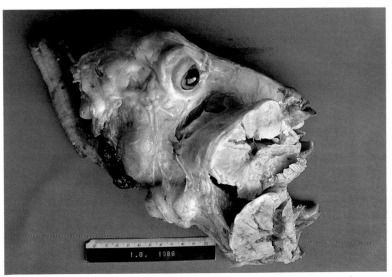

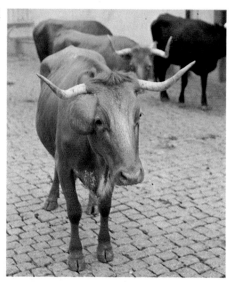

**31 Neoformation – head:
cow** A subcutaneous round and
firm tumour extends to the right
side of the head, from the base of
the horn up to the eye. The adjacent
lymph nodes were not enlarged and
the rectal temperature was normal.

Hypothetical diagnosis: Neoplasia;
abscess.

Decision: Slaughter authorized
with special precautions.

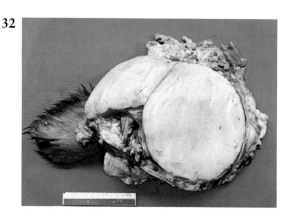

32 Fibrolipoma – neoplasia: cow Neoplasia
shown in the previous picture. The cut surface
revealed an homogeneous, smooth and shining
surface, yellow-orange in colour and greasy to
touch.

Decision: Approval with elimination of the
tumour (post-mortem).

24

33 Neoplasia – horn: ox The left horn was replaced by a neoplasia, the size of a football, hard and crusty, with extensive congestive haemorrhagic areas.

Hypothetical diagnosis: Neoplasia.

Decision: Slaughter authorized with special precautions.

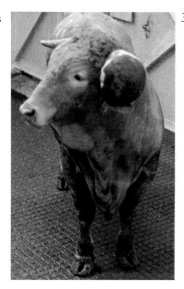

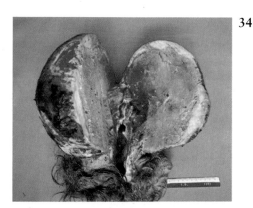

34 Osteosarcoma – horn: ox Section of the neoplasia shown in the previous picture. The cut surface was solid, hard, highly congested and with some superficial blood clots.

Decision: Total condemnation.

35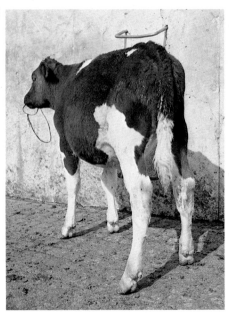

35 Acute meteorism (tympanism) – left flank: calf Young calf with marked swelling of the left flank, the typical depression of that area having disappeared. The facies was anxious, the limbs apart and the animal looked frequently at the flank.

Decision: Authorization for slaughter delayed.

36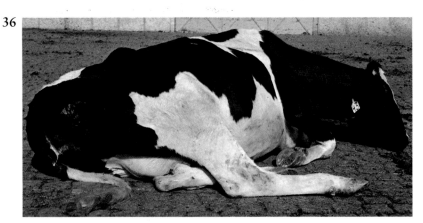

36 Purulent vulvar discharge: cow This recumbent prostrated cow, with sad facies, presented a yellow-green vulvar discharge, with the characteristics of purulent exudate.

Hypothetical diagnosis: Suppurative metritis.

Decision: Authorization for slaughter delayed.

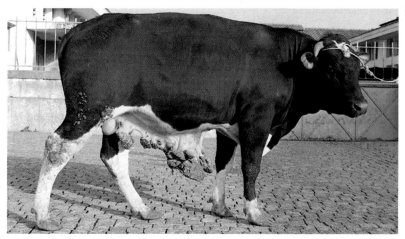

37 Papillomatosis – prepuce: ox Multiple tumours, consistent and with cauliflower appearance were distributed along the prepuce.

Decision: Slaughter authorized under special precautions. The tissue removed for histopathological examination should be collected both from the base of the tumour and from its surface.

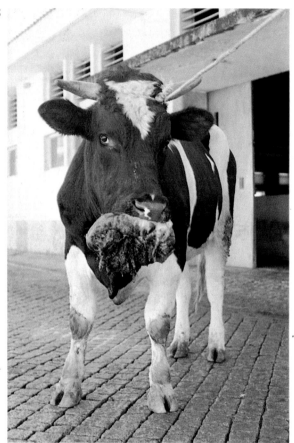

38   Basal cell carcinoma – lower lip: ox   The lower lip was totally replaced by a very large, cauliflower-like neoplasia, with firm consistency and areas of congestion and haemorrhage.

Decision: Condemnation at the ante-mortem inspection.

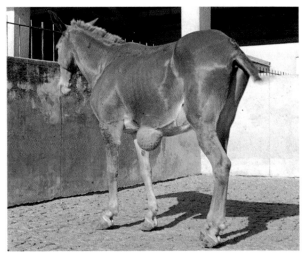

39 Tumefaction – abdominal wall: horse
Subcutaneously in the abdominal region, near the external
thoracic vein, a round swelling the size of a melon could be
seen. Palpation showed it had soft consistency, was non-
deformable and painless.

Hypothetical diagnosis: Neoplasia; cyst; Haematoma;
Hernia.

Decision: Slaughter authorized with special precautions.

**40 Myxoma –
tumefaction:
horse** The cut
surface of the
neoplasia shown in
the previous picture
revealed it had an
heterogeneous
appearance.

Decision: Approval
with elimination of
the neoplasia
(post-mortem).

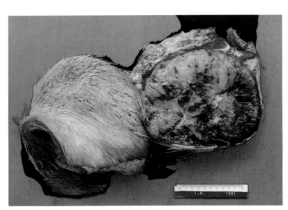

Emergency slaughter

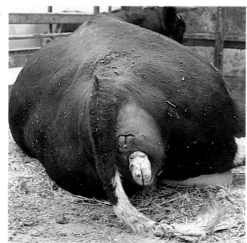

41   Dystocia: cow   This cow had started giving birth 2 days before being admitted for emergency slaughter. It had moderate tympanism and a rectal temperature of 40.6°C.

Decision: Authorization for slaughter delayed.

42   Compound fracture – metacarpus: mule   A compound fracture of the right thoracic limb was observed in this mule. The animal was apyretic.

Decision: Slaughter was authorized under special precautions. In emergency slaughter the degree of bacterial contamination must be determined and antibiotics detected in the meat and kidneys. Antimicrobial products are detected and identified by studying growth inhibition of special microbial strains in special culture medium. A piece of muscle of approximately 70 g and a fragment of kidney of approximately 30 g were used for tests.

Inspection criteria:
(a) Detection negative in the muscle and viscera – approval.
(b) Positive detection in the muscle or viscera – totally condemned for human consumption, because in such cases the bacteriological examination is not conclusive.

2: The carcase – bones, muscles, joints, tendons and ligaments

**43 Fatigued meat – carcase:
cattle** Emaciated carcase, showing a brownish colour.

Boiling test: 2.2 ml. Final pH of the longissimus dorsi muscle = 6.6.

Decision: Total condemnation. Fatigued meat often has an apple-like odour; when cooked it is dry, tough and tasteless.

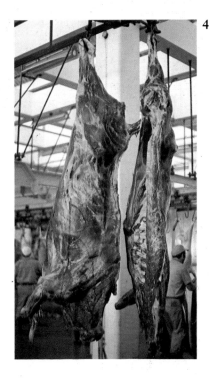

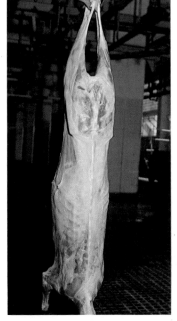

44 Hydrocachexia – carcase: sheep
Reduced subcutaneous fat, generalized muscle atrophy and anaemia. The skeleton can be seen under the musculature. The superficial tissues had a moist appearance and there was dripping from the inner area of the thighs.

Decision: Total condemnation.
The carcase also presented hydropic atrophy of the perirenal and heart fat and also of the fat surrounding some lymph nodes (superficial cervical and prefemoral).

31

45

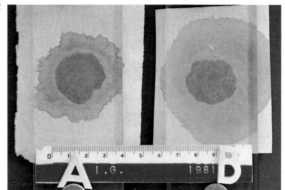

45 Measurement of the free water in the meat
Two measurements of free water in homologous muscle fragments (0.5 g), carried out between two compressing glass slides over filter paper, treated with a saturated solution of potassium chloride.

Test A: Normal – the ratio between the diameter of the aqueous stain and the meat stain is inferior to 2 (50: 25.5).

Test B: High water content – the ratio between the diameter of the aqueous stain and the meat stain is higher than 2 (67: 25.5).

Decision: Total condemnation in B. A proportion can also be established between the areas of the two types of stains with more accurate results.

46

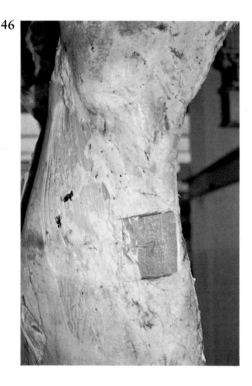

46 Zenker's degeneration – carcase: cattle The musculature was pale yellow, resembling fish muscle.

Differential diagnosis: Haemolytic anaemia; Nutritional anaemia; Hyaline muscular dystrophy.

Decision: Total condemnation.

47 Zenker's degeneration – carcase: cattle The muscle fragment on the left is from the carcase shown in **46**. The fragment on the right is from a normal homologous muscle.

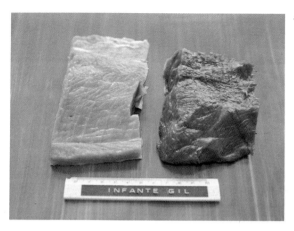

48 Presternal calcification – carcase: cattle In the fibrous and fat tissues of the brisket, at the level of the first and second ribs, an area of dystrophic calcification was found. The calcified material was softened and drained out of the cut surface.

Differential diagnosis: Abscess.

Decision: Approval with elimination of the calcified tissues.

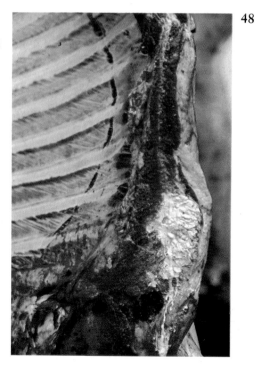

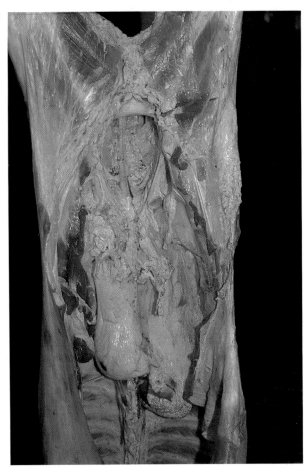

49   Focal fat necrosis – carcase (fat): sheep   The flank, perirenal and pelvic fat showed numerous dry milky-white necrotic foci, clear distinct from the surrounding normal fat.

Decision: Total condemnation.

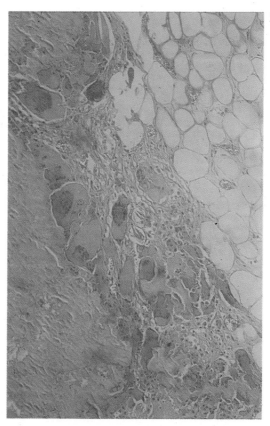

50 Necrosis of the abdominal fat – perirenal fat: sheep The changes occurring in the fat determined a reaction of macrophages leading to the formation of giant cells. Alcohol and xylene did not dissolve the altered fat contrasting to what happened with the normal fat. H. & E.

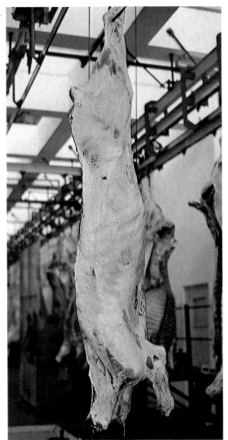

51 Gelatinous oedema – carcase: cattle Carcase showing reduced muscular development and pale colour. There was little subcutaneous fat which looked abnormally wet and shiny, giving the carcase a pale hyaline appearance.

Decision: Total condemnation. The kidneys were equally discoloured, indicating the existence of a general systemic reaction.

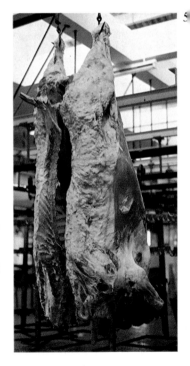

52 Adipoxanthosis (carotenosis) – carcase: cattle Carcase of an old animal with golden-yellow highly developed subcutaneous fat. Results of the Remington-Fournier tests:
(a) detection of carotinoid pigments: positive;
(b) detection of biliary pigments: negative.

Decision: Approval.

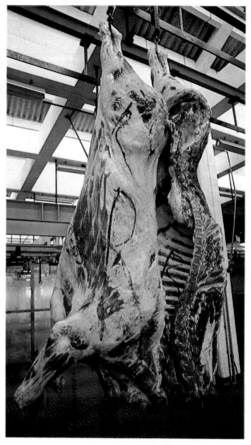

53 Icterus (jaundice) – carcase: cattle   The fat was yellow-green as were the aorta and ligament of the neck. During refrigeration the abnormal colour intensified.

Differential diagnosis: Adipoxanthosis; Impregnation by picric acid, atabrine or trypaflavine.

Decision: Total condemnation.
The Herlich and Remington-Fournier tests for the detection of biliary pigments were positive. Blood-free samples of perirenal fat and sinovial fluid must be collected to perform the tests.

54

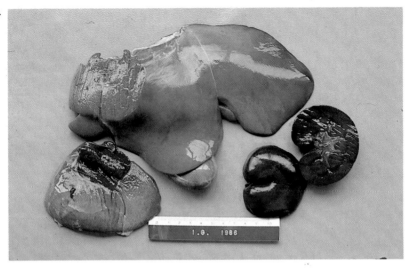

55

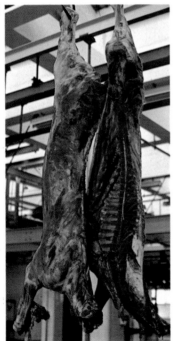

54 Lesions – viscera: sheep *Liver:* slightly hypertrophic and pale due to acute hepatitis lesions with predominance of degenerative changes of the hepatic cells. *Kidney:* the dark brown colour of the organ, whose capsule was easily removed, corresponded to a cholaemic nephrosis. *Spleen:* The organ was hypertrophic with softened consistency of the pulp which showed a very dark red colour in a case of haemorrhagic inflammation.

Decision: Total condemnation.
Note: The viscera were removed from an animal with haemolytic jaundice, which developed subsequent to vaccination.

55 Xanthomatosis – carcase: horse The subcutaneous fat showed an abnormal dark brown colour.

Decision: Total condemnation.

56 Xanthomatosis – carcase: horse Detail of the abnormal fat shown in 55.

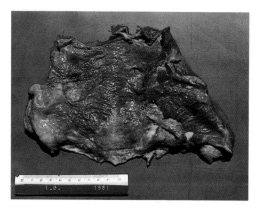

57 Abnormal subcutaneous fat – carcase: cattle The only post-mortem change detected was the abnormal golden-yellow colour of the entire fat, of a gelatinous consistency.

Laboratory analysis: Ratio of iodine in the fat = 50.9.

Decision: Approved for human consumption as inferior meat.

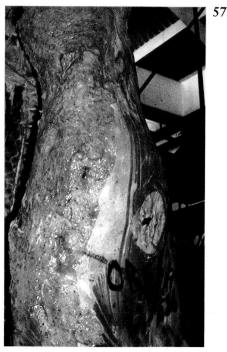

58

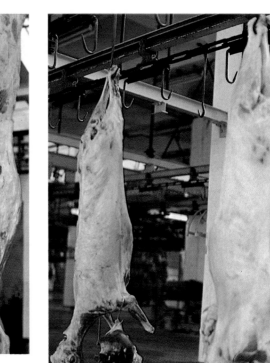

58 Abnormal subcutaneous fat – carcase: cattle The subcutaneous fat was abnormally pale and moist. Acute generalized lymphadenitis and thyroid hypertrophy were also noticed.

Laboratory test: Water content of the longissimus dorsi muscle: 78.2%.

Decision: Total condemnation.
The detection of thyreostatic substances (methylthiouracil) in the meat yielded positive results (*see* **424** and **827**).

59 Feverish meat – carcase: sheep The carcase on the left showed congestion of the superficial vessels and the subcutaneous fat and connective tissue were yellow-pink. Degenerative changes were found in the liver and kidney. This was a typical case of feverish meat.

Differential diagnosis: Incomplete bleeding; Aseptic hyperthermia.

Decision: Total condemnation.

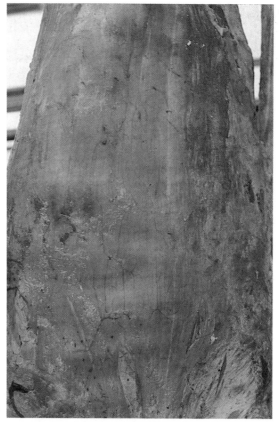

60 Feverish meat – carcase: cattle Detail of a carcase showing dark red musculature and ectasia of the small subcutaneous blood vessels. These changes are characteristic of carcases from animals slaughtered during a fever syndrome.

Differential diagnosis: Insufficient bleeding. Hyperthermia due to effort (aseptic).

Decision: Total condemnation.

61

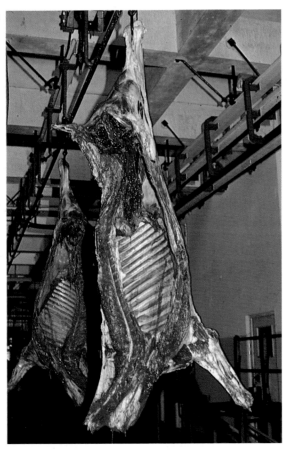

61   Traumatic lesions in the soft tissue of the hip – carcase: horse   The hindquarters, especially in the lumbar region and hip showed extensive haemorrhages. At the evisceration a considerable haemoperitoneum was found. The animal had slipped while running and fell with his posterior limbs wide open. Following this type of accident animals may present with subnormal rectal temperature due to internal haemorrhage.

Decision: Approval after elimination of the affected tissues.

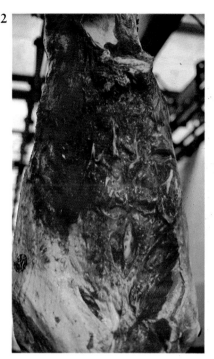

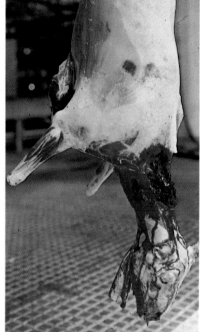

62 Recent generalized traumatic lesions – carcase: cattle Extensive muscular laceration could be noticed, together with haemorrhages and intermuscular and subaponeurotic oedema.

Decision: Total condemnation.

63 Laceration of the neck – carcase: sheep The dorsal tissues of the neck were extensively destroyed due to savaging by a dog. Slaughter immediately followed the accident after approval at the ante-mortem inspection.

Decision: Approval after extensive elimination of the wounded tissues plus the immediately surrounding ones.

International institutions, for example FAO/OMS recommended the following actions: If the aggression took place 2 days before slaughter, approval of the ante-mortem and post-mortem inspections are indicated, with elimination of the affected tissues plus the surrounding ones. Slaughter may be suspended for a quarantine period of 8 months following contact.
In both cases the professional risks that a suspicion of rabies involves have to be considered. The inspector should not limit his action to measures related to the suspicion of rabies. Other pathological problems have to be considered according to each case.

64

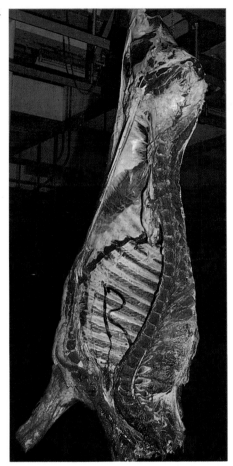

64 Necropurulent bursitis – withers: cattle After the splitting of the carcase a necropurulent inflammatory reaction was noticed in the withers. The yellow-grey creamy pus was odourless and the regional lymph nodes were reactive.

Decision: Total condemnation.

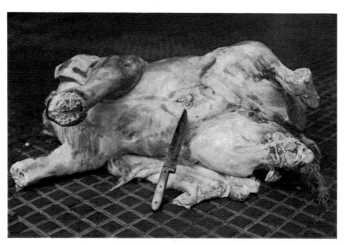

65 Omphalophlebitis – carcase (navel): calf An infection of the umbilical cord caused a septicopyohaemia with metastatical abscesses in the knee joint (purulent arthritis).

Decision: Total condemnation.

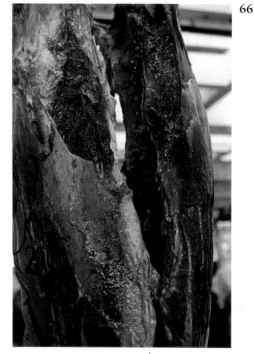

66 Necrotic exudative dermatitis – carcase (abdominal wall): cattle The dark brown abdominal wall showed a marked oedema, had a greasy feel, a foul smell and cloudy exudate. It easily disintegrated by palpation and showed gaseous crepitation.

Decision: Total condemnation.

67

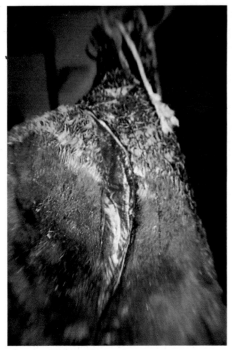

**67   Black leg (symptomatic anthrax) –
carcase: posterior limb cattle**   The incision
of a subcutaneous swelling and underlying
muscles revealed an acute inflammatory
reaction with congestion and exudation of
serous, bloody fluid. Crepitation of rancid
smelling gas was noticed.

Decision: Total condemnation.

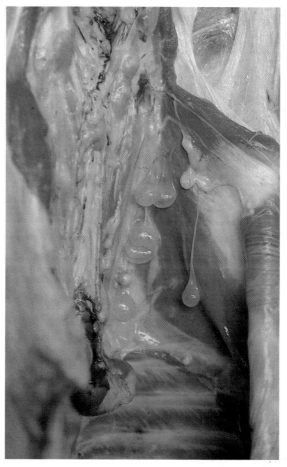

68 Cysticercosis – carcase: sheep Numerous pediculated vesicles, with a clear content similar to water, could be seen in the peritoneal cavity in a case of infection by *Cysticercus tenuicollis*.

Decision: Approval with elimination and destruction of the cysts and infected parts.
Total condemnation is justifiable when the animals are emaciated or if the disease had severe adverse effects on the general condition of the carcase.

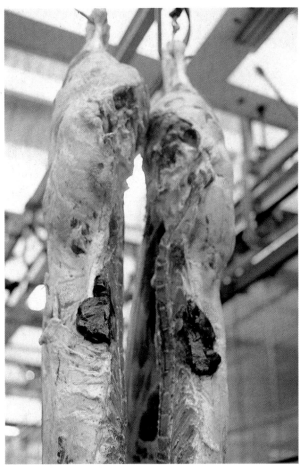

69 Melanotic sarcoma – carcase: cattle During
skinning, a solid neoplastic mass was noticed in the
subcutaneous connective tissue in the dorsolumbar region.
It was black and presented the characteristics of the
malignant melanotic tumours.

Decision: Total condemnation.

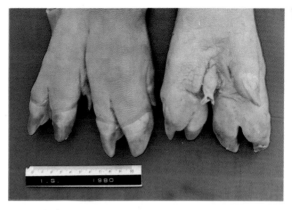

70 Polydactylism – feet: swine Symmetrical duplication of the fingers of the anterior limbs.

Decision: Approval with elimination of the feet.

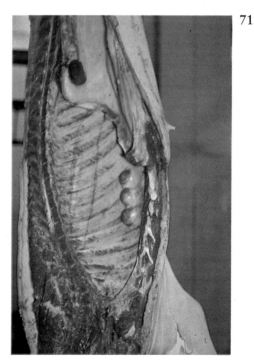

71 Nodular swellings – ribs: swine The alignment of the nodules in three consecutive ribs and their clear limits favoured the diagnosis of bony callus.

Hypothetical diagnosis: Bony callus; Osteosarcoma.

72

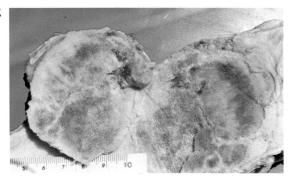

72 Bony callus – rib: swine The incision of the nodules shown in the previous picture exposed a bony callus. The cut surface was granular and homogeneous and the blood irrigation evenly distributed.

Decision: Approval with elimination of the bone lesions.

73

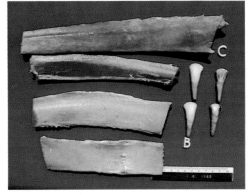

73 Depigmentations – fragments of ribs and incisor teeth: cattle The picture shows the contrast in colour between normal (B) and reddish (C) fragments of homologous ribs and incisor teeth. The red pigment was thought to be due to feeding with dye-producing plants (alizarine).

Differential diagnosis: Osteohaemochromatosis; Porphyria; Lymphoblastic lymphosarcoma (metastasis).

Decision: Approval with elimination of the skeleton.

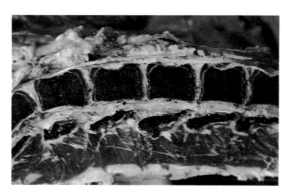

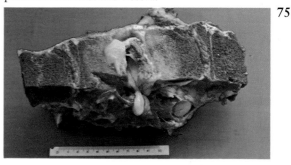

74   Osteohaemochromatosis – fragment of vertebral column: cattle   The vertebrae were stained dark-red, almost black, both in the body and processes, due to abnormal pigment metabolism. The kidneys showed a similar colour.

Decision: Approval with elimination of the affected parts in the carcase and viscera.

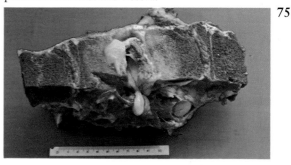

75   Purulent osteitis – fragment of vertebral column: cattle   At the splitting of the carcase a suppurative infection was noticed in the vertebral column. One vertebra and the corresponding intervertebral disc were affected, becoming partially destroyed. A viscous yellow pus filled the resulting space.

Bacteriological examination of the pus: This showed *Clostridium histolyticum.*

Decision: Total condemnation.

76

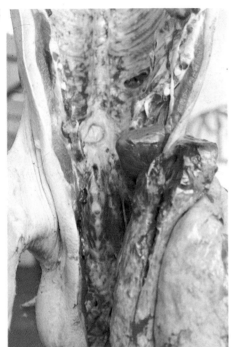

76 Fibropurulent osteitis – dorsal vertebra: swine A suppurative infection of a dorsal vertebra almost destroyed it completely. The pus was yellow and creamy. Microbial embolism had occurred in the pulmonary diaphragmatic lobe which displayed a focal inflammatory lesion. Bacteriological examination of the pus showed *Escherichia coli.*

Decision: Total condemnation.

77

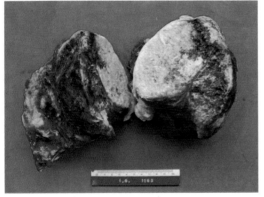

77 Chronic osteitis – ischiatic tuberosity: cattle The hypertrophy of the ischiatic tuberosity resulted from a chronic inflammatory reaction subsequent to a fracture.

Differential diagnosis: Neoplasia.

Decision: Approval with elimination of the affected tissues.

78 Osteolytic osteitis – femur: cattle The femur showed a osteolytic osteitis of the condyles. This condition is frequently bilateral.

Decision: Approval with elimination of the affected tissues.

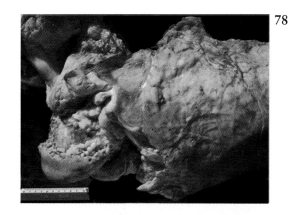

79 Tuberculosis – vertebrae: cattle Circular osteal erosions containing yellow, caseous necrotic material were found in the vertebrae, and in other organs and tissues.

Decision: Total condemnation. If tuberculosis is confined to a single bone lesion, only the skeleton need be discarded.

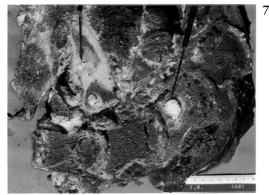

80 Actinomycosis – head (macerated skull): cattle Actinomycosis is a specific inflammatory disease, caused by a microorganism and characterized by opposing reactions in the bone: osteolytic osteitis and, simultaneously, new bone formation from the periosteum, ossifying periosteitis.

Decision: Approval if no other lesions are found, with elimination of the head and tongue.

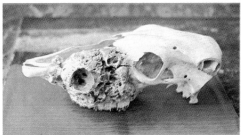

81

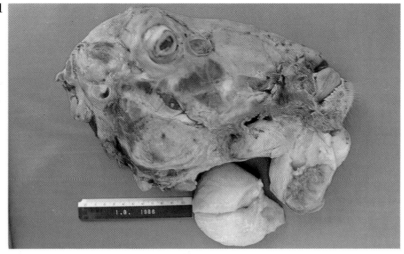

82

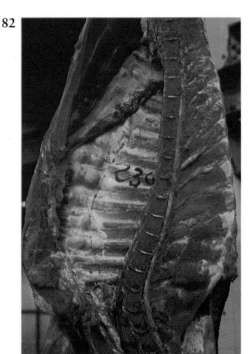

81   Hard fibroma – lower jaw: sheep   A whitish tumour with a well-defined outline adhered to the right lower jaw. When sectioned, the consistency was hard and the cut surface had a pink tone.

Differential diagnosis: Actinomycosis; Keloid.

Decision: Approval with elimination of the head.

82   Osteosarcoma – ribs: cattle Several nodules had arisen from the ribs and showed a distinct invasive growth towards the costal cartilage in the sixth and seventh ribs.

Differential diagnosis: Bony callus.

Decision: Total condemnation.

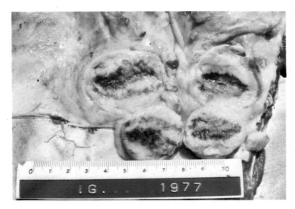

83 Osteosarcoma – ribs: cattle Incision of the
nodules in the previous picture was easy and revealed an
internal structure of cartilage at the periphery and small
calcium deposits in the centre, together with congestive
and haemorrhagic foci.

Differential diagnosis: Fracture.

Decision: Total condemnation.

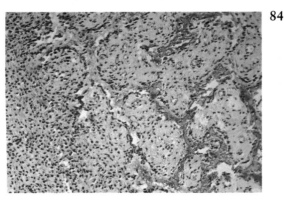

84 Osteosarcoma – rib: cattle The structure of
the Haversian system was clearly reproduced in the
neoplastic tissue. Some areas were becoming
calcified. H. & E.

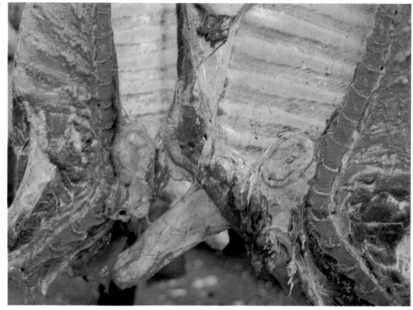

85 Fibrosarcoma – rib: cattle In the thorax, at the first rib, a neoplasia was found slightly larger than a fist, well adherent to the neighbouring tissues and yellowish-pink in colour. The histological diagnosis was fibrosarcoma.

Differential diagnosis: Neurofibroma; Thymus.

Decision: Total condemnation.

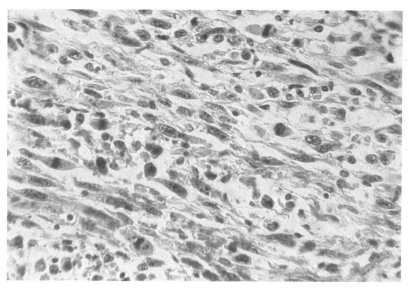

86   Fibrosarcoma – rib: cattle   Highly malignant tumour, characterized by atypical cells and high number of mitoses. H. & E.

87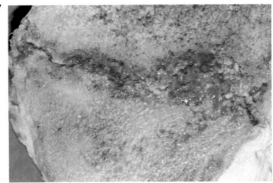

87 Fibrochondro-osteosarcoma – rib: cattle
An incised rib tumour with granular lardaceous appearance and a central core where loss of substance had occurred together with congestion and haemorrhage.

Differential diagnosis: Fracture.

Decision: Total condemnation.

88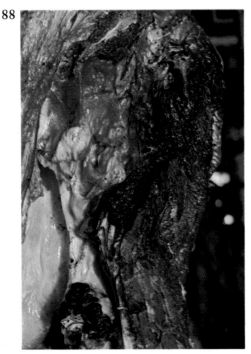

88 Melanotic tumour – sacrum: horse A bright black pigment was noticed in the sacral vertebrae at the splitting of the carcase. It was a melanotic tumour.

Decision: Total condemnation.

89 Metastasis of carcinoma – ribs: horse Numerous small irregular white-pink nodules could be seen on the parietal pleura. The incision showed a lardaceous appearance typical of neoplasias. Two of the ribs also presented well-limited rounded swellings corresponding to the bone localization of the same tumours.

Differential diagnosis: Tuberculosis; Actinobacillosis.

Decision: Total condemnation.

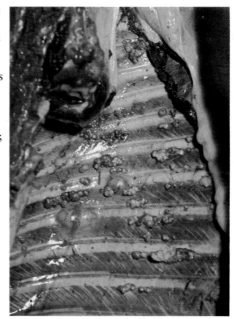

90 Metastasis of lymphoblastic lymphosarcoma – ribs: cattle Across the parietal pleura some prominent swollen dark-red ribs could be seen. The incision, easily accomplished with a knife, denuded a granulous and highly haemorrhagic tissue.

Differential diagnosis: Porphyria; Osteohaemochromatosis.

Decision: Total condemnation.

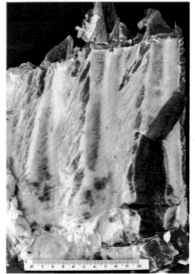

91

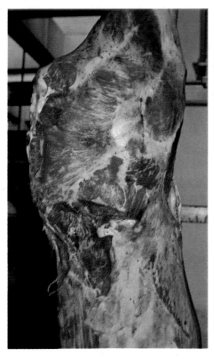

91 Lipomatosis (pseudohypertrophia lipomatosa) muscles: cattle The buttock muscles were hypertrophic and highly consistent justifying an exploratory incision that revealed an abnormal muscle with fibres in which the normal tissue had been replaced by fat and by fibrous connective tissue.

Differential diagnosis: Muscular dystrophy; chronic myositis; leukosis.

Decision: Approval with elimination of the affected muscles.
When the process is generalized total condemnation should be applied.

92

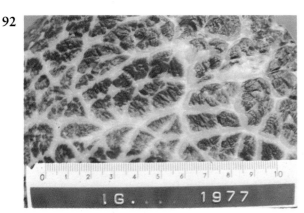

92 Lipomatosis (pseudohypertrophia lipomatosa) – muscle: cattle Transverse section of the muscle showing the muscular bundles separated by white-yellow trabeculae of fat and connective tissue in variable amounts. A fragment of this muscle floated in water, releasing small drops of fat.

93 Atrophy – muscles: cattle The musculature was atrophic with concave profiles and outstanding bone prominences.

Decision: Approval with elimination of the atrophic hindquarter.

The atrophic muscles were thin, yellow-pink and flaccid. This situation is usually related to inactivity due to problems in the bones or joints and also to changes in the nerves, tendons or fibrous sheaths of tendons. The final pH of such meat is sometimes higher than 6.0, due to the tiredness of the animal.

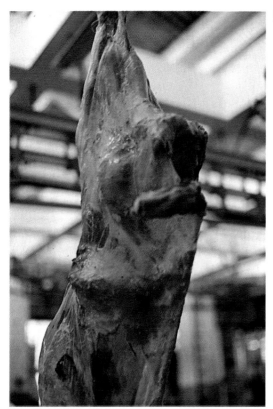

94 Zenker's degeneration – muscle: cattle The muscle's unstained area, with the appearance of fish muscle, corresponded to Zenker's degeneration of the fibres.

Differential diagnosis: Toxic myopathy.

Decision: Approval with elimination of the affected muscle.

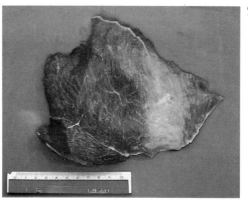

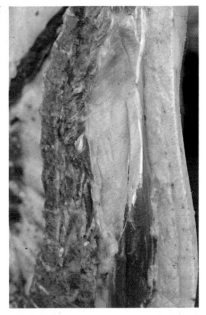

95 Pale soft exudative (PSE) – muscle: swine After splitting it was noticed that the longissimus dorsi muscle looked pale, flaccid and exudative, in clear contrast with the other muscles.

Differential diagnosis: Zenker's degeneration; toxic myopathy.

Decision: Approval with elimination of the affected muscle.
PSE: Criteria at post-mortem inspection.
(a) Total condemnation in generalized and extremely intense cases of PSE.
(b) Approval as inferior meat in cases of medium or mild intensity. (c) Approval without restrictions in very mild cases.
(d) Partial condemnation in cases where only few muscles are affected, with their elimination.

96 Pale soft exudative (PSE) – muscle: swine The semitendinosus muscle was paler than usual, appearing abnormally moist due to exudation. The fibres were also excessively separated.

Decision: Approval with elimination of the affected muscle.
The muscles in which PSE is more expressive are: longissimus dorsi, semi-tendinosus, deep pectoral and gluteus medius. In suspicious cases they must be carefully examined. Whenever possible, the inspector should delay judgement for 24 or 48 hours, to check changes in the meat's organoleptic characteristics, which are susceptible to decrease or increase over time.

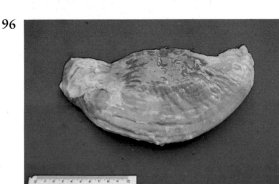

97 Multiple haemorrhages – muscle: cattle All muscles in the carcase showed multiple haemorrhages of various sizes and shapes, making it look unpleasant (splashing of the musculature).

Decision: Total condemnation. The haemorrhages were caused by fear felt by the animal at the moment of slaughter. Premature putrefaction of the meat frequently occurs in these cases.

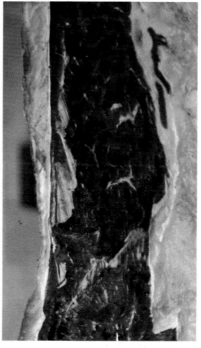

98 Inflammatory reaction – muscle (hip): cattle A limited swelling in the hip detected ante-mortem, was shown at post-mortem to be a 'cystic' formation, limited by connective tissue and inserted between the regional muscles. It contained numerous small pieces (B and C) of variable size, shape and colour, which seemed to arise from small granular structures located in the cyst's inner wall. The histological examination showed they were fibrin, surrounded by a delicate fibrous capsule. The regional lymph nodes were not reactive.

Decision: Approval with elimination of the affected tissues.

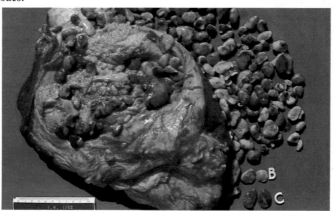

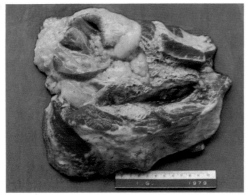

99 Degenerative necrotic myositis – muscle: cattle The muscles of the neck were affected by a necrotic and degenerative process, which could be due to an intramuscular injection.

Decision: Approval with elimination of the affected muscles.

100 Chronic myositis – muscle: cattle The striated muscle showed reasonably extensive areas of chronic inflammation with replacement of the muscle by fibrous connective tissue, which gave it hard consistency and a whitish-yellow colour.

Differential diagnosis: Zenker's degeneration; Neoplasia.

Decision: Approval with elimination of the affected tissues.

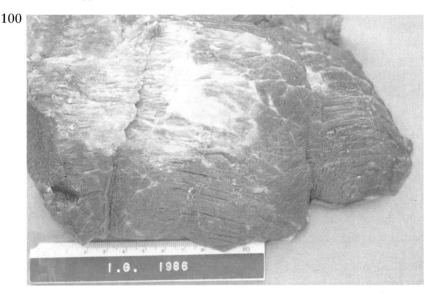

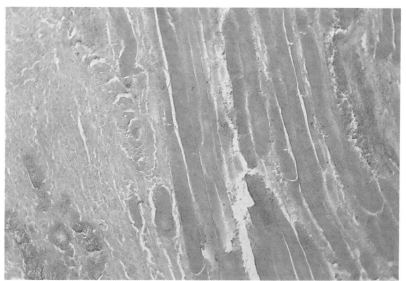

101 Chronic myositis – muscle: cattle Degenerative or necrotic process of the muscle fibres, which in some areas showed dystrophic calcification. The tissue was progressively replaced by connective tissue. H. & E.

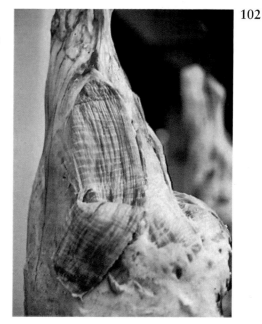

102 Eosinophilic myositis – posterior limb: cattle The muscles of the thigh looked green, showing a clear transverse striation of the fibres, which appeared excessively delineated.

Differential diagnosis: Putrefaction.

Decision: Total condemnation. Further areas in the musculature showed similar characteristics of eosinophilic myositis. Section of the lymph nodes revealed an equally greenish colour (infiltration of eosinophils).

103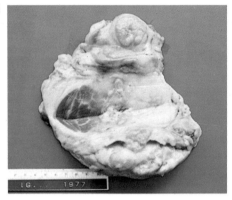

103 Actinobacillosis – muscle: cattle Incision of the swollen masseter revealed several granulomas, bulging from the cut surface, surrounded by connective tissue and with variable amounts of yellow pus in the centre. The regional lymph nodes were not reactive.

Differential diagnosis: Non-specific abscesses.

Decision: Approval with elimination of the head and tongue.

104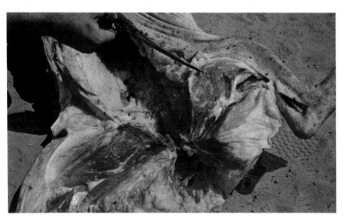

104 Cysticercosis – muscle: swine The incision of the adductor muscles of the thigh revealed several vesicular ovoid nodules, whitish-yellow and smaller than a green pea. They were larvae of *Taenia solium.*

Differential diagnosis: Sarcocystosis; Trichinosis; Calcified microfoci of myositis; Toxoplasmosis.

Decision: Total condemnation.
In cases of moderate or small infection (infestation) the judgement can be conditionally approved to the freezing of the carcase, which has to be maintained at −10°C. for 25 days. Some authors believe this is not a safe way to destroy the cysticerci, advising instead salt curing the meat. The Commission of the Codex Alimentarius, in its Code, CAC/RCP 34–1985, indicates total condemnation in cases of heavy infection. The number of cysticerci to be regarded as heavy infestation shall be determined by the responsible authority. In cases of moderate or small infestation (infection) the thermal treatment (Kf) is recommended if the heat treatment option is taken to 60°C. (140°F.) in the centre of the meat.

105 Trichinosis – muscle: swine
Trichinoscopical image of a formalin fixed muscle, showing several cysts of *Trichinella* (*Trichinella spiralis*).

Differential diagnosis: Sarcosporidiosis; Cysticercosis; Calcified microfoci of myositis; Toxoplasmosis.

Decision: Total condemnation. The samples for trichinoscopical examination are removed from the diaphragm crura (at least one sample per crus), tongue, masticator muscle, or abdominal muscles, the size of a walnut.

106 Lymphoblastic lymphosarcoma – muscle (diaphragm): cattle Areas of abnormal pale muscle were noticed in the diaphragm, associated with a well-defined tumorous growth. When the diaphragm was sectioned the muscle fibres appeared separated by a yellowish tissue.

Differential diagnosis: Lipomatosis; Chronic myositis.

Decision: Total condemnation.

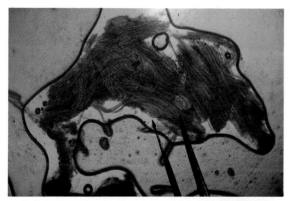

105

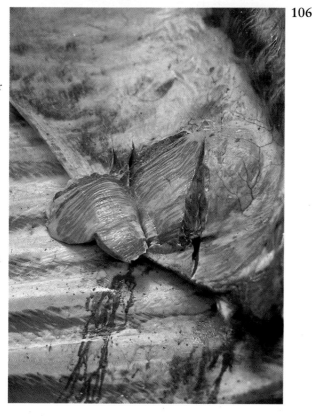

106

107

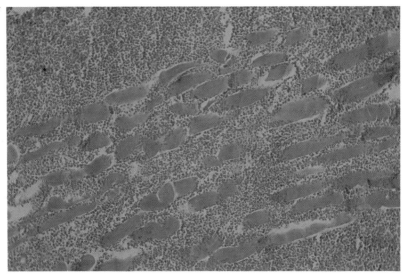

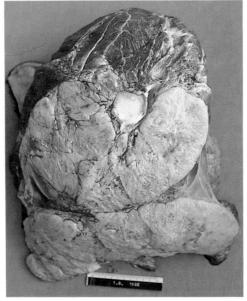

107 Leukosis – muscle (diaphragm): cattle A cellular population of mature lymphocytes was found to dissociate and break up the fibres of the striated muscle of the diaphragm, in a case of lymphocytic leukosis in an adult bovine. H. & E.

108 Rhabdomyosarcoma – muscle: cattle Neoplasia of yellowish colour, developed from the muscles of the shoulder, leading to the destruction of the neighbouring tissues.

Differential diagnosis: Chronic myositis; Lipomatosis.

Decision: Total condemnation.

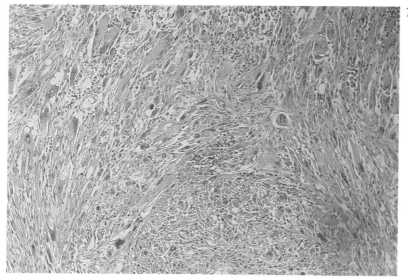

109 Rhabdomyosarcoma – striated muscle: cattle Neoplasia characterized by the large number of atypical cells and numerous images of cell division, revealing its high malignancy. H. & E.

110 Inflammatory reaction – brisket: cattle An unspecific inflammatory reaction developed in the brisket region, probably traumatic and characterized by a fibrinous exudate and small necrotic foci.

Decision: Approval with elimination of the affected tissues.

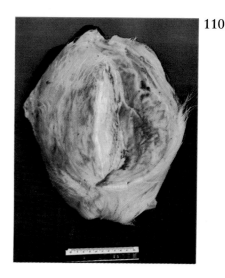

110

111

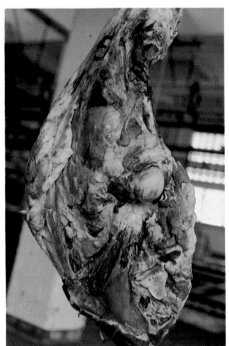

111 Bone taint – posterior limb: cattle The soft tissues around the hip joint exhaled a putrid smell. They showed a grey-greenish colour and the consistency was slightly softened. The aetiology of bone taint is not clearly established. Possibly enzymatic problems and microbial contamination (anaerobics) are at its origin.

Decision: Total condemnation. This case was noticed in a refrigerated carcase, 24 hours post-slaughter.

112

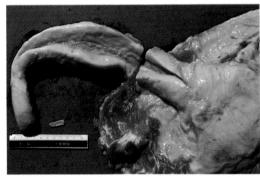

112 Fistula – costal wall: cattle In the inner face of the costal wall a firm white cord of fibrous tissue was noticed, which after incision was seen to have a central lumen. At the extremity a small lamellar piece was found. It was a fistula formed by the migration of a foreign body.

Differential diagnosis: Neurofibromatosis.

Decision: Approval with elimination of the newly formed and affected tissues.

113   Soft fibroma – anterior limb: cattle   A bizarrely shaped tumour was attached to the soft tissues of the forearm by a pedicle. Its consistency was similar to muscle, light-brown and partially surrounded by connective tissue.

Decision: Approval with elimination of the neoplasia.

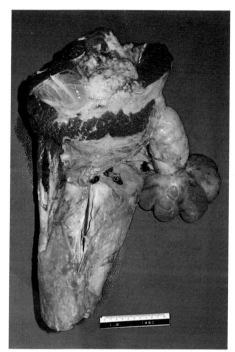

113

114 and 115   Arthritis – knee joint: horse Massive swelling of the knee joint (**114**). The incision showed it to be due to the accumulation of a serous-fibrinous exudate in the joint cavity (**115**). The inner surface of the swelling also showed fibrinous inflammatory reaction.

Differential diagnosis: Purulent arthritis; Arthrosis.

Decision: Approval with elimination of the affected tissues. The Codex Alimentarius Commission, in its Code, recommends the following criteria at the post-mortem inspection: (a) Non-infectious arthritis: approval with elimination of the affected tissues. (b) Acute infectious arthritis (fibrinous, purulent), for example, polyarthritis in newborn

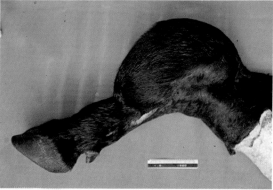

114

115

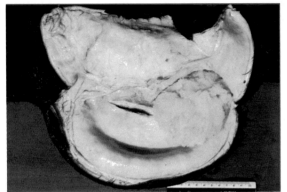

animals – total condemnation or approval with elimination of the affected parts of carcases, subject to the results of the laboratory examination.
(c) Chronic arthritis – approval with elimination of the affected parts of the carcase.

116

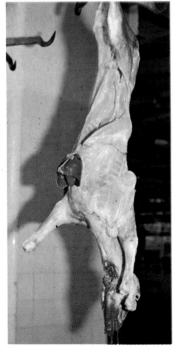

116 Purulent arthritis – knee joint: sheep A purulent inflammatory reaction was present in this animal's left carpal joint. The homolateral axillary lymph node was considerably swollen and numerous small abscesses (pyoemicro abscesses) were found in the liver, as a consequence of haematogenous dissemination.

Decision: Total condemnation.

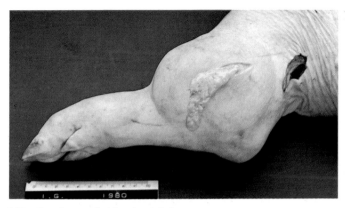

117 Purulent arthritis – hock joint: swine An acute
inflammatory reaction in the hock joint led to considerable local
swelling due to the accumulation of viscous pus, containing many
yellow granules.

Decision: Total condemnation.

118

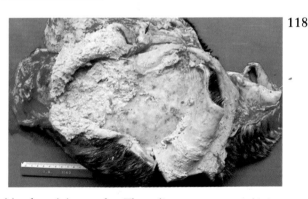

118 Tuberculous arthritis – knee joint: cattle The radiocarpometacarpal joint
was substantially thickened due to tuberculous lesions. The local exploratory
incisions revealed abundant inodorous yellow necrotic material. The regional
lymph nodes were also involved. The picture shows the connective tissue
surrounding the joint with multiple red stained areas and the covering skin with
small caseocalcified nodules or tubercles.

Decision: Total condemnation.
The various decisions suggested for tuberculous lesions will be found in the Code,
CAC/RCP 34–1985, of the Commission of the Codex Alimentarius.

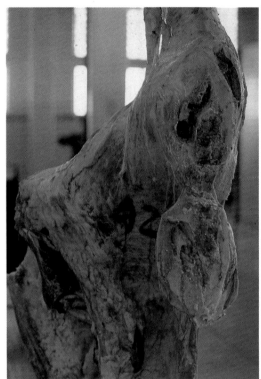

119 Actinomycosis - stifle joint: cattle Stifle joint tumour, which showed after incision to be due to an actinomycotic process with osteolysis, necrosis of the bone and involvement of the soft surrounding tissues.

Differential diagnosis: Neoplasia.

Decision: Approval with elimination of the affected tissues.

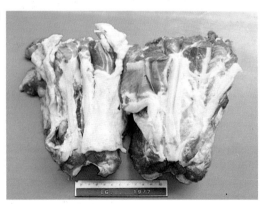

120 Icterus (jaundice) – ligament of the neck: sheep The difference in colour between two identical pieces of meat, which include the ligament of the neck surrounded by the neck dorsal muscles. The example on the right is from a normal animal, and on the left from a sheep with jaundice.

Decision: Total condemnation (case of jaundice).

121 Necropurulent ulceration - tendo achillis (t. calcaneous communis): cattle A necrotic lesion occurred in the hock, affecting the Achilles tendon. The popliteal lymph node was markedly reactive.

Decision: Approval with elimination of the affected limb, subject to laboratory examination.
Cases such as this demand a laboratory examination.

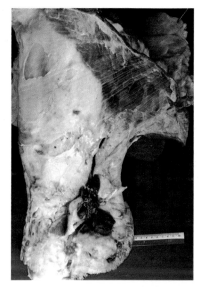

122 Chronic inflammatory reaction – ligament of the neck: cattle Numerous cord-shaped masses, fibrous and pearly white were arising from the ligament of the neck. Their calibre was very homogeneous. The microscopical examination confirmed the fibrous nature of these structures which seemed to be part of a chronic inflammatory reaction.

Decision: Approval with elimination of the affected tissues.

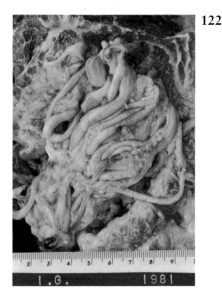

3: The integumentary system: skin and appendages

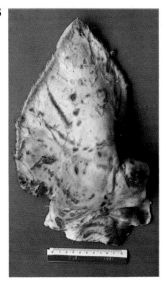

123   Traumatic lesions – auricle: swine
These usually arise from accidents due to aggression from companions during transport or a period of rest in the lairage.

Decision: Approval with elimination of the auricle.

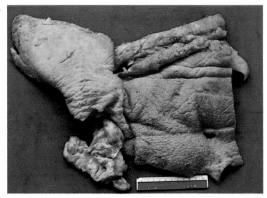

124   Acute dermatitis – fragment of skin and lymph nodes: swine   The skin was reddened with a granular appearance. Purulent lymphadenitis could be seen in the mandibular, superficial linguinal and prefemoral lymph nodes.

Differential diagnosis: Allergic dermatitis; Erythema of erysipelas.

Decision: Total condemnation.

125 Chronic dermatitis – skin (carcase): swine

The skin was markedly red due to generalized inflammatory hyperaemia of parasitic aetiology. The lymph nodes were not reactive.

Differential diagnosis: Erythema of erysipelas; Allergic dermatitis; Sunburn dermatitis.

Decision: Approval with elimination of the skin and feet.

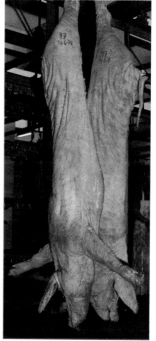

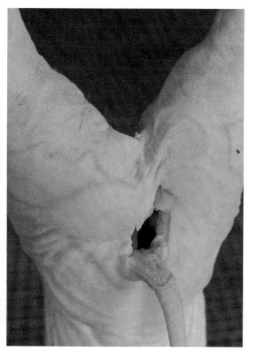

126 Chronic dermatitis – skin (carcase): swine

Thickening of the skin caused by hyperplasia of the connective tissue, typical of chronic dermatitis; the concentrically disposed red streaks suggested a fungal aetiology, which was not possible to confirm because the hair had been removed by scalding.

Decision: Approval with elimination of the skin.

127

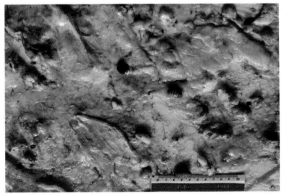

127 Warbles (hypodermosis) – hide: cattle The subcutaneous tissue showed the presence of small regular cavities and nodules produced by *Hypoderma* larvae which could actually be seen.

128

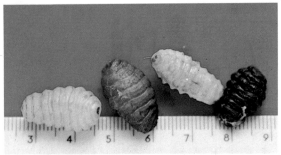

128 Hypoderma larvae: cattle

**129 Besnoitiosis (globidiosis) –
aponeurosis (thoracic limb): cattle**
Numerous small hard granules, looking
like sand, could be seen in the
aponeurosis of the thoracic limb. They
were *Globidium besnoiti* cysts.

Differential diagnosis: Cysticercosis.

Decision: Approval with elimination of
the affected tissues. In cases of generalized
infection total condemnation is
recommended.

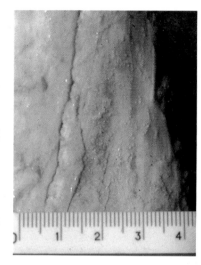

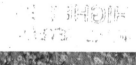

130 Cutaneous leukosis – skin: cattle
The skin showed multiple hairless
nodules, slightly prominent, the diameters
varying from 1 to 3 cm. Histological
examination confirmed the
lymphosarcomatous nature of the lesions.

Differential diagnosis: Sporotrichosis;
Nodular dermatitis.

Decision: Total condemnation.

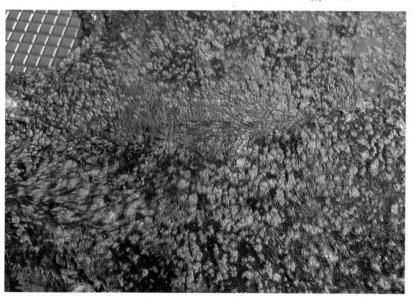

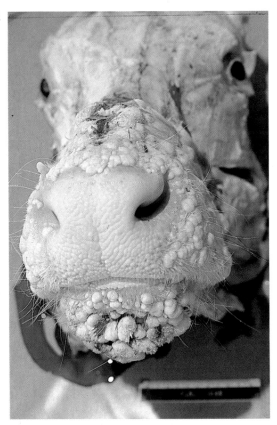

131 Papillomatosis – head skin: cattle In the skin covering the lower lip, and in the hairless area of the muzzle up to the nostrils, multiple pedicellated masses could be seen, frequently assuming a typical cauliflower appearance. These corresponded to a large number of papillomas, benign tumours developed from the malpighian epithelium.

Differential diagnosis: Nodular dermatitis; Epitheliomas; Mycosis.

Decision: Approval with elimination of the head and tongue.

132

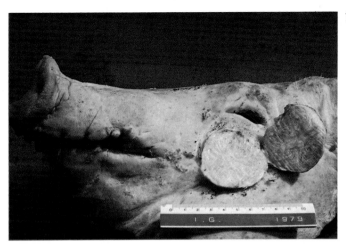

132 Fibroma – skin (face): swine   The cut surface of a round, well-limited and firm infraorbital neoplasia is shown. Its colour was white and it had a fasciculated appearance.

Decision: Approval with elimination of the neoplasia.

133

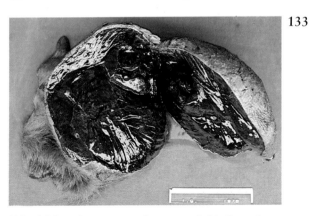

133 Melanotic sarcoma – fragment of skin from the neck: cattle   Subcutaneously, in the left side of the neck, a voluminous ovoid and firm neoplasia was located, whose cut surface was black and shiny.

Decision: Total condemnation.

134

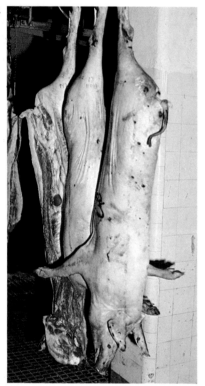

134 Malignant cutaneous melanosis – skin (carcase): swine In several areas of the skin small spherical protruding black nodules were located. The mandibular lymph nodes were swollen and equally black.

Differential diagnosis: Pigmentary lesions in the lymph nodes due to feeding with cork oak nuts.

Decision: Total condemnation.

135 Spindle cell sarcoma – skin: cattle Large numbers of white or pink neoplasias of variable size could be seen in the skin covering the lower jaw and throat. They were prominent and lardaceous.

Differential diagnosis: Hyperkeratosis; Non-specific granulomas; Papillomatosis.

Decision: Total condemnation.

135

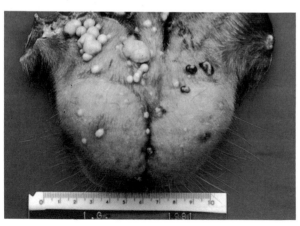

136

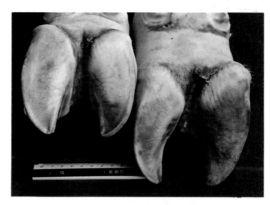

136 Foot and mouth disease – feet: cattle The inspection of the feet revealed the presence of an acute inflammatory reaction in the hoof crown, with hyperaemia and a few scabs. A more detailed examination showed identical lesions in the interdigital grooves and also in the tongue, lips and rumen.

Decision: Total condemnation based on the complete set of lesions.

137

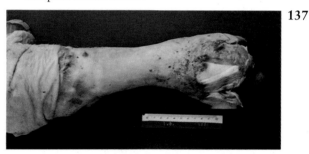

137 Chronic inflammatory reaction – foot: swine The distal extremity of a limb showed a hard tumefaction consisting of fibrous tissue as a result of a chronic inflammatory reaction.

Differential diagnosis: Neoplasia.

Decision: Approval with elimination of the affected foot.

138

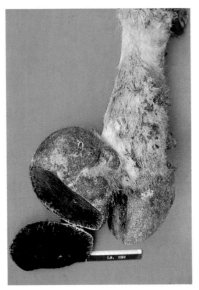

138   Benign melanoma – limb: cattle
A spherical neoplasia developed from the shank's skin. Incision showed it to be black.

Differential diagnosis: Malignant neoplasias.

Decision: Approval with elimination of the affected extremity.

139

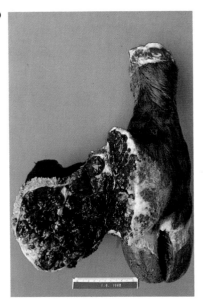

139   Undifferentiated cell sarcoma – limb: cattle   A lardaceous and highly congested neoplasia was attached to the animal's shank. Its hyperaemia made it look extremely dark, nearly black.

Differential diagnosis: Melanoma.

Decision: Total condemnation.

140 Fibrosarcoma – foot: cattle A neoplasia located in the extremity of the limb led to the destruction of the hoof. Incision showed it to be formed of a white fibrous tissue.

Differential diagnosis: Chronic inflammatory reaction.

Decision: Total condemnation.

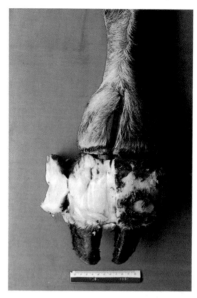

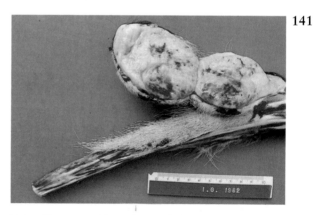

141 Fibroma – tail: cattle A globular growth, which arose from the dermal connective tissue, having a whitish-yellow tissue with few haemorrhages.

Differential diagnosis: Fibrosarcoma.

Decision: Approval with elimination of the neoplasia.

142

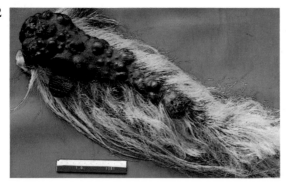

142 Malignant melanoma – tail: horse A large number of small round swellings could be noticed under the skin at the root and inferior face of the tail. Their sizes were variable and they were black and shiny which identified them as melanotic neoplasias.

Decision: Total condemnation.

143

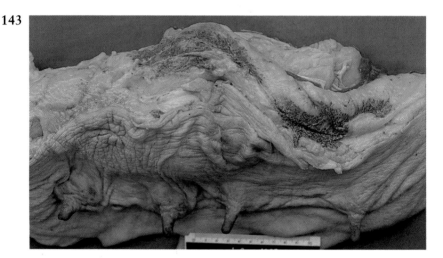

143 Melanosis – udder: sow The incision of the linea alba during evisceration disclosed an almost black tissue, which proved to be present in several mammary glands.

Decision: Approval with elimination of the mammary glands and affected tissues.

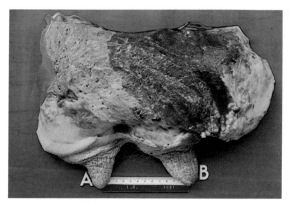

144　Abnormal colour – mammary gland: cow　The complete hindquarter of the udder (B) showed a brown colour suggesting a pathological problem. However, microscopic examination did not show any disturbance. Consequently, the possibility of the intramammary injection of a coloured product to suspend lactation was admitted. The superficial inguinal lymph node was normal.

Decision: Approval with elimination of the udder.

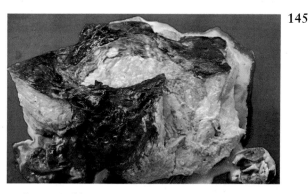

145　Perimammary haemorrhages – udder: cow　In the course of dressing an intense external haemorrhage was noticed between the skin and the tissues around part of the udder. No lesions were seen in the mammary gland itself; therefore, the haemorrhage was thought to be due to traumatism. The superficial inguinal lymph node, although reddened due to the presence of blood, was not reactive.

Differential diagnosis: Mastitis.

Decision: Approval with elimination of the udder.

146

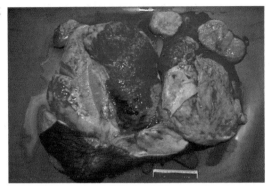

146 Traumatic mastitis – udder: cow An extensive area of the udder presented intense red colour due to recent haemorrhage, probably traumatic. Some blood clots can be seen distal to the haemorrhage.

Decision: Approval with elimination of the udder.

147

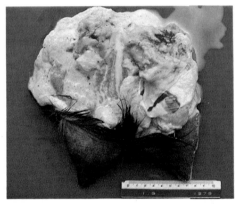

147 Purulent mastitis (brucellosis) – udder: goat The udder was bilaterally swollen with subcutaneous oedema, in the midst of which gas bubbles of unidentified origin were seen. At the incision of the mammary gland a liquid similar to milk was produced. Purulent foci were located in the parenchyma of the gland.

Decision: Total condemnation.

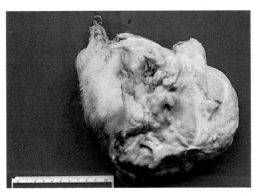

148 Necropurulent mastitis – udder: ewe The udder shown in the picture was hypertrophic and abnormally firm, especially in some restricted areas. The incision showed a necrotic and purulent inflammation.

Decision: Total condemnation.

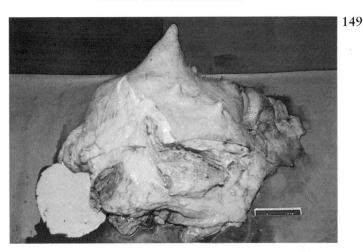

149 Necropurulent mastitis – udder: cow A marked increase in the size of the udder was noticed and the covering skin was distended by the accumulation of liquified purulent material which drained from the incision.

Decision: Total condemnation.

150

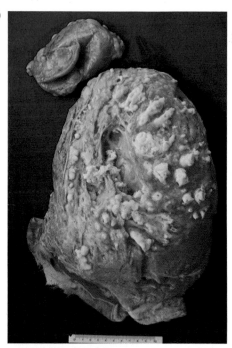

150 Necropurulent mastitis – udder: cow The palpation of the udder had revealed that some areas were highly consistent. The incision showed that yellow necrotic and purulent material was present in the glandular tissue. The corresponding lymph nodes were swollen, moist and congested.

Decision: Total condemnation.

151

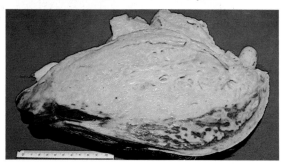

151 Necrotic mastitis – udder: cow The incision of an abnormally firm quarter showed oedema of the subcutaneous tissue and intense inflammatory reaction of a restricted area of the mammary gland, in which necrotic yellow foci, together with congestion and haemorrhages, were noticed. The lactiferous sinus, ducts and remaining glandular tissue were unaffected.
Bacteriological examination of the lesion showed *Staphylococcus aureus*.

Decision: Total condemnation.

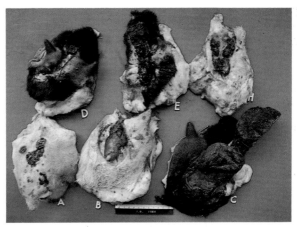

152 Gangrenous mastitis – udders: ewe   Several animals of the same consignment were equally affected, showing necrotic areas in the udder with considerable loss of tissue.
Bacteriological examination of the lesion showed *Pseudomonas fluorescens* and *Staphylococcus aureus*.

Decision: Total
condemnation.

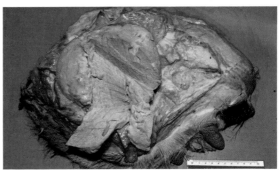

153 Sequestrum – udder: cow   The incision of an abnormal quarter revealed a spherical mass of necrotic tissue, looking like boiled tissue, surrounded by a pasty viscous material.
Its clear isolation from the normal gland suggests that a circulatory disturbance might have originated this problem.

Differential diagnosis: Neoplasia.

Decision: Approval with elimination of the udder.

154

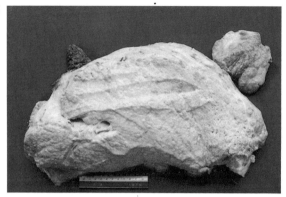

154 Chronic mastitis – udder: cow   The gland was slightly atrophic and excessively firm. The cut surface was finely granular, interrupted by strands of white fibrous tissue.

Differential diagnosis: Neoplasia; actinobacillosis.

Decision: Approval with elimination of the udder.

155

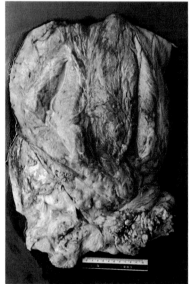

155   Caseous tuberculous mastitis – udder: cow   The incision of the udder showed caseocalcified nodules isolated or in small groups. In the mucosa of the teat and lactiferous sinus the nodules were more abundant. There was a breakdown of body resistance.

Differential diagnosis: Non-specific mastitis.

Decision: Total condemnation.

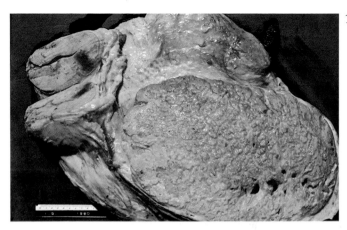

156 Infiltrative caseous tuberculosis – udder: cow The incision of a highly consistent udder showed caseous necrosis. A few interspersed areas of lardaceous tissue were also seen. In the corresponding lymph node caseating necrosis was also present. This set of lesions was thought to be part of a breakdown of body resistance.

Differential diagnosis: Necropurulent mastitis.

Decision: Total condemnation.

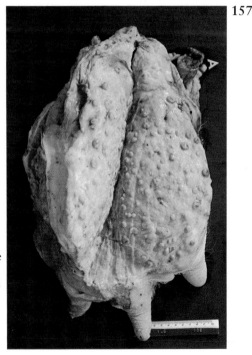

157 Actinobacillosis – udder: cow The incision of an excessively firm udder showed numerous raised granules which were visible under the covering skin. In the centre of the nodules a sulphur-yellow pus, typical of actinobacillosis, was seen. The lymph nodes were not reactive.

Differential diagnosis: Neoplasia; Tuberculosis; Chronic mastitis.

Decision: Approval with elimination of the udder.

158

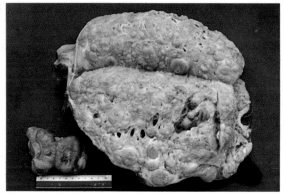

158 Actinobacillosis – udder: cow Most of the glandular parenchyma was destroyed by the specific granules surrounded by fibrous tissue. The prominence of the nodules from the cut surface is considered typical of this affection. The lesion was extensive to the lymph nodes.

Differential diagnosis: Neoplasia; tuberculosis; chronic mastitis.

Decision: Total condemnation.

159

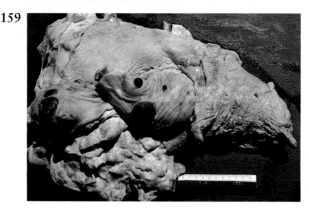

159 Actinomycosis – udder: sow The skin of the udder showed brown circular scabs and palpation revealed moderately free nodules. Incision uncovered necropurulent lesions. The lymph nodes were not reactive and did not show actinomycotic lesions.

Differential diagnosis: Non-specific purulent mastitis; Neoplasia.

Decision: Approval with elimination of the complete udder.

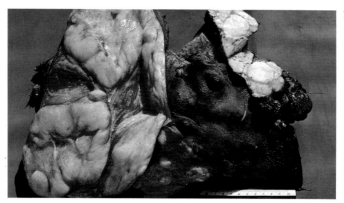

160 Fibromatous neoplasias – udder: mule Firm nodules of variable sizes were located in the mammary gland. Incision showed a smooth cut surface, light yellow and shiny.

Differential diagnosis: Malignant neoplasias; Actinobacillosis.

Decision: Approval with elimination of the udder.

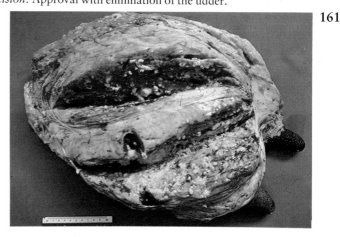

161 Purulent mastitis (malignant evolution) – udder: cow The palpation of the hypertrophic udder showed a granular structure. The incision revealed purulent foci. The pus, more or less consistent, was yellow-green.

Examinations:
(a) histopathological: this showed purulent mastitis with signs of cancerous evolution.
(b) bacteriological: this showed *Corynebacterium pyogenes*.

Decision: Total condemnation.

162

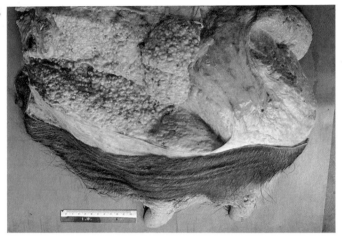

162   Adenoma (malignant evolution) – udder: cow   Large areas of the gland were replaced by a granular tissue, prominent at the cut surface.

Differential diagnosis: Chronic mastitis; Tuberculosis; Actinobacillosis.

Decision: Total condemnation.

163

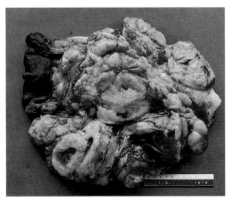

163   Fibrosarcoma – udder: mare   A light yellow neoplasia, of ill-defined limits, was found near the mammary gland.

Decision: Total condemnation.

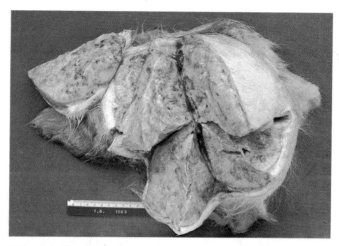

164   Spindle cell sarcoma – udder: cow   A tumefaction located in one quarter of the udder was seen to correspond to a malignant tumour with yellow cut surface and numerous focal haemorrhages.

Differential diagnosis: Mastitis.

Decision: Total condemnation.

4: The digestive system

The head

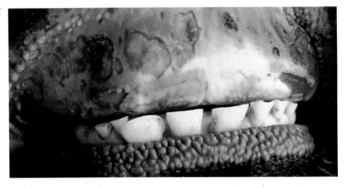

165 Ulcerative cheilitis – upper lip: cattle The irregular ulcers in the upper lip, with a more or less congestive base, were the result of the destruction of the epithelium by the foot and mouth disease virus.

Differential diagnosis: Vesiculous stomatitis; Mucosal disease; Rinderpest; Traumatic cheilitis; Muzzle disease.
The cheilitis illustrated above is part of a group of lesions of foot and mouth disease (type C virus) (*see* **182** and **356**).

Decision: Total condemnation.

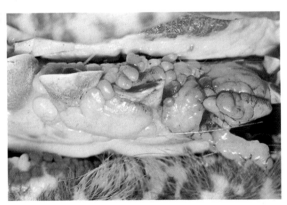

166 Epulis – gums: cattle In the gum of the lower jaw, around the incisor teeth there is a proliferative multinodular process; the pinkish, shiny tissue bleeds easily.

Decision: Approval with elimination of the head and tongue.

167 Keloid – mandible: horse A hard tumorous growth, 10.5 cm in diameter, attached to the lower jaw. The cut surface was white and shiny, with focal haemorrhages. It was a chronic inflammatory lesion, formed by fibrous tissue. These frequently recur after surgical excision.

Decision: Approval with elimination of the affected tissues.

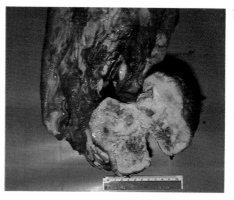

167

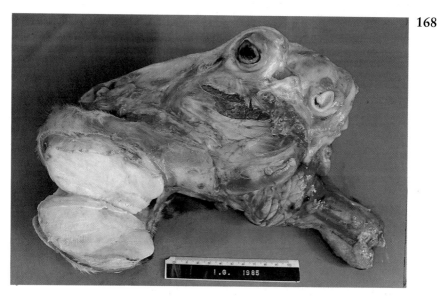

168

168 Haemangiopericytoma – lower jaw: sheep A tumour, larger than a lemon, adheres to the soft tissues of the lower jaw. At palpation a soft consistency was noticed at the surface, becoming harder in the inner areas. The cut surface was white and smooth.

Decision: Approval with elimination of the affected tissues.

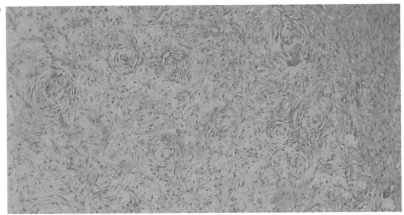

169   Haemangiopericytoma – lower jaw: sheep   The tumour originated from the submandibular region and showed a cellular arrangement in concentric layers, some of which had a central lumen. H. & E.

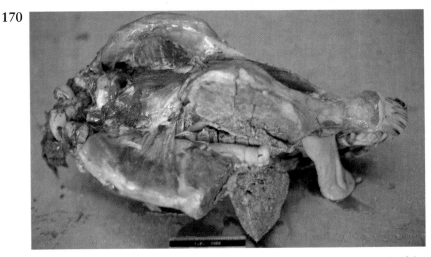

170   Undifferentiated cell carcinoma – mandible: horse   The left branch of the mandible was considerably swollen. The incision showed that the consistency was softened, as the osteal tissue had been replaced by a solid reddish neoplastic growth.

Decision: Total condemnation.

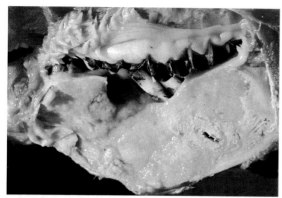

171 Spindle cell sarcoma – lower jaw: sheep The left lower jaw was affected by a destructive neoplasia. The dental alveoli have been destroyed and several teeth are missing. There is a focus of secondary infection in the central area of the neoplasia, and greenish-yellow pus.

Differential diagnosis: Suppurative osteitis; Infected fracture.

Decision: Total condemnation.

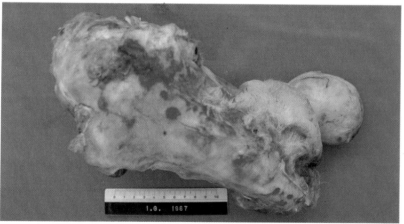

172 Spindle cell sarcoma – upper jaw: sheep Ante-mortem examination showed a globular swelling, 6 cm in diameter, covered by unchanged skin, which developed in the soft tissues of the mandible. The removal of the skin showed that the neoplasia was attached to the mandible by a pedicle. The cut surface was regular, smooth, shiny and pinkish.

Decision: Total condemnation.

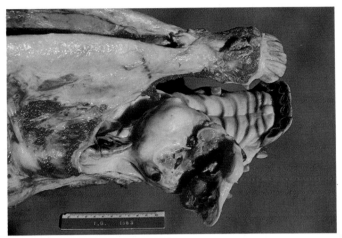

173 Fibrosarcoma – palate: horse A globular, bosselated mass arose from the palate. The neoplasia, of variable consistency, presented a heterogeneous cut surface, either gelatinous and fibrous or bony.

Decision: Total condemnation.

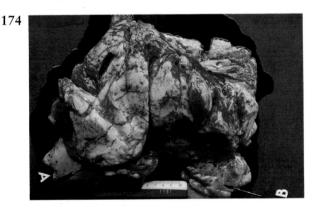

174 Chronic inflammatory reaction – mandibular salivary gland: cattle The submandibular gland was thickened due to abnormal development of fibrous tissue. The typical pink tone was replaced by a whitish-yellow colour with numerous haemorrhages. B: mandibular lymph node.

Differential diagnosis: Neoplasia.

Decision: Approval with elimination of the affected organ.

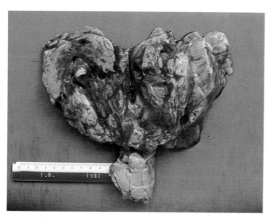

175 Adenocarcinoma – mandibular salivary gland: cattle The salivary gland, clearly hypertrophic, was congested and presented several haemorrhagic foci. In areas where the normal appearance of the organ was changed the consistency was firm.

Differential diagnosis: Inflammatory reaction.

Decision: Total condemnation.

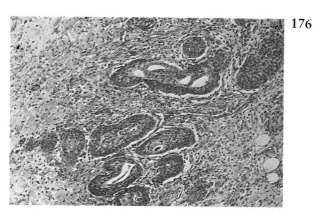

176 Adenocarcinoma – salivary gland: cattle The cords of neoplastic cells show a clear tendency to form tubular structures. H. & E.

177

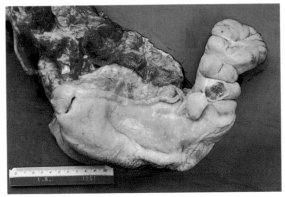

177   Malformation – tongue: horse   A succession of
grooves of variable depth give the tongue a
multilobulated appearance, particularly in the anterior
end. There was a considerable amount of connective
tissue infiltrating the muscle fibres.

Decision: Approval with elimination of the tongue.

178

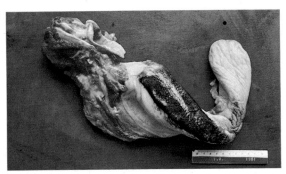

178   Impregnation of dye – tongue: horse   A dull
black colour on the posterior surface of the tongue.
Small superficial cuts were noticed and the incision
revealed that the abnormal colour was limited to the
epithelium.

Differential diagnosis: Melanotic neoplasia.

Decision: Approval with elimination of the tongue.

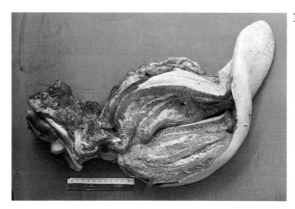

179 Pseudohypertrophia lipomatosa – tongue: cattle
The tongue was uniformly hypertrophic. The incision
showed the presence of large amounts of connective
tissue and fat in between the muscular fibres.

Decision: Approval with elimination of the tongue.

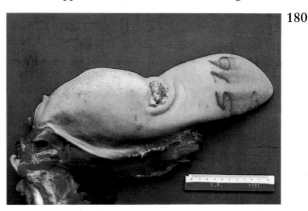

180 Traumatic ulcer – tongue: cattle   This traumatic
lesion in front of the dorsal prominence of the tongue
was caused by blunt particles in the food, namely awns.
These lesions often become the site of entry for various
pathogens.

Decision: Approval with elimination of the tongue.

181

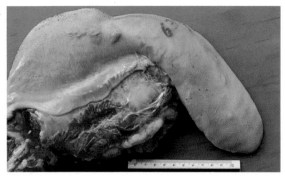

181   Aphthous glossitis – tongue: cattle   Patches of epithelium are raised on the tongue surface due to the accumulation of fluid between the cells of the epithelial stratum spinosum. These lesions are characteristic of vesiculous evolution of foot and mouth disease.

Decision: Total condemnation.

182

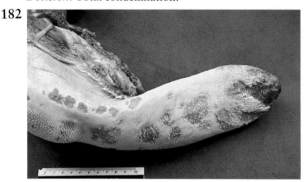

182   Necrotic ulcerative glossitis (foot and mouth disease) – tongue: cattle   Several healing ulcers on the surface of the tongue corresponded to a late stage in the evolution of vesicular lesions. This is typical of foot and mouth disease (type C virus) (*see* **165** and **356**).

Differential diagnosis: Necrobacillosis.

Decision: Total condemnation.
The Code, CAC/RCP 34–1985, of Codex Alimentarius Commission recommends: (a) in normally free or nearly free countries: total condemnation of carcase and viscera; (b) in other countries or areas the decision to be in accordance with prevailing animal health measures consistent with effective public health protection; particular attention must be paid to secondary bacterial infections and general findings, and there must be effective measures to prevent contamination of abattoirs.

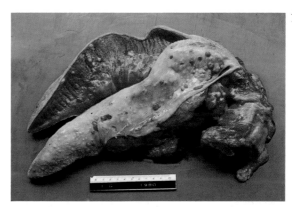

183 Actinobacillosis – tongue: cattle At the dorsum and both sides of the tongue there are numerous red nodules and small raised patches. Yellow nodules, typical of actinobacillosis, are also present.

Differential diagnosis: Non-specific granulomas.

Decision: Approval, with elimination of the tongue.

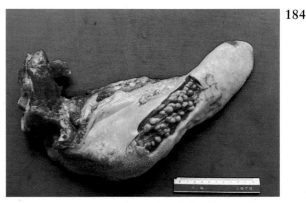

184 Actinobacillosis – tongue: cattle A series of small nodules are present within the tongue, after removal of the superficial epithelium, in which numerous discrete raised patches had already been noticed. Such nodules contained an elastic yellow pus with small bright yellow granules.

Decision: Approval, with elimination of the tongue.

185

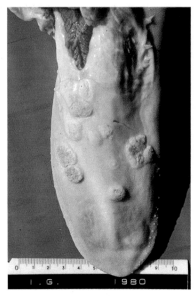

185 Papillomatosis – tongue: cattle
Well-defined and flat cauliflower-shaped
nodules, in the ventral face of the tongue.
They were benign tumours which arise
from the malpighian epithelium, supported
by a delicate vascularized connective
stroma.

Differential diagnosis: Actinobacillosis;
Necrobacillosis; Malignant neoplasia.

Decision: Approval with elimination of the
tongue.

186

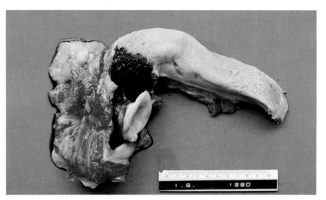

186 Melanotic carcinoma – tongue: swine At the base of
the tongue and in the tissues around the epiglottis is a black
shiny tissue with the features of malignant neoplasia,
developed from melanin-producing cells.

Differential diagnosis: Infiltration of dye.

Decision: Total condemnation.

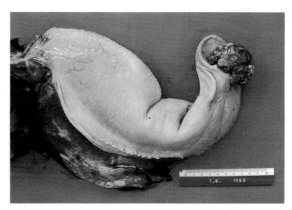

187 Squamous cell carcinoma – tongue: cattle In the ventral face of the tongue near the free anterior end, a pedicellated neoplasia, reddish and lobulated, bleeding easily.

Differential diagnosis: Papilloma; Actinobacillosis.

Decision: Total condemnation.

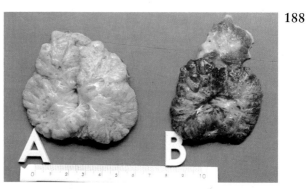

188 Congestive haemorrhagic amygdalitis – tonsils: cattle The normal tonsils (A) clearly contrast with (B), which are congestive and haemorrhagic.

189

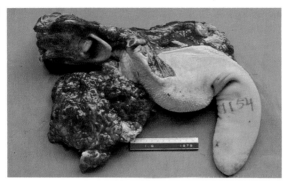

189 Carcinoma – pharyngeal tonsil: cattle At the
back of the mouth, adherent to the pharynx, there is a
soft neoplasia. The tumour contains mixed yellow and
red areas, the last ones corresponding to congestion and
haemorrhages.

Decision: Total condemnation.

190

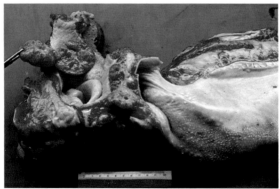

190 Spindle cell carcinoma – pharynx: cattle An egg-
sized mass adheres to the pharynx by a short pedicle.
This neoplasia was nearly covering the entrance to the
oesophagus and the larnyx. It showed a smooth and
silky cut surface, highly congested.

Decision: Total condemnation.

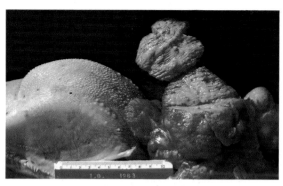

191   Actinobacillosis – pharynx: cattle   A pediculated
mass, at the back of the tongue, was, at incision, highly
fibrous. Several prominent nodules of actinobacillosis a
few millimetres in diameter, and containing yellow pus,
were present.

Differential diagnosis: Tumour of the tonsils.

Decision: Approval with elimination of the affected
tissues.

Oesophagus and stomach

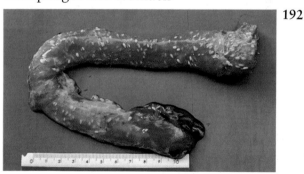

192   Sarcosporidiosis – oesophagus: sheep   White
and roughly elliptical nodules underneath the adventitia
of the oesophagus. They were larvae of *Sarcocystis*
without surrounding inflammatory reaction.

Decision: Approval with elimination of the oesophagus.

193

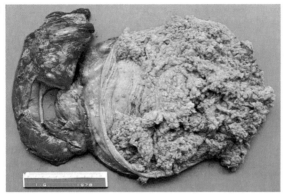

193 Papillomatosis – oesophagus: cattle Incision of swelling in the middle third of the oesophagus revealed numerous villous, benign tumours.

Decision: Approval with elimination of the oesophagus.

194

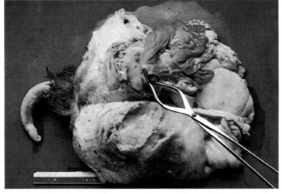

194 Hernia – abomasum: cattle During the removal of the skin a swelling of the prepuce, already noticed in the ante-mortem inspection, was identified as a ventral hernia of the abomasum, which was enclosed in a sheath of fibrous inflammatory tissue.

Decision: Approval with elimination of the affected tissues.

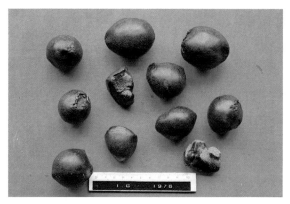

195 Egagropilus – rumen: sheep   Spherical, ovoid and elliptical dark brown bodies with a smooth shiny surface, were found in the rumen of a sheep. Some were broken and showed an irregular surface. In one, the central core comprised a tangle of hair covered by a hard mineral shell and coloured by vegetable pigments.

Decision: Approval (elimination of the egagropilus).

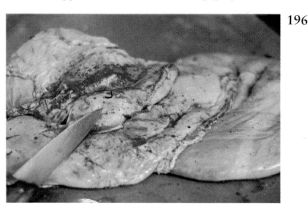

196 Reticuloperitonitis – reticulum: cattle   A traumatic reticuloperitonitis was caused by a wire that could be seen crossing the reticulum wall, in which it determined a serofibrinous local inflammatory reaction.

Decision: Approval with elimination of the forestomachs.

197

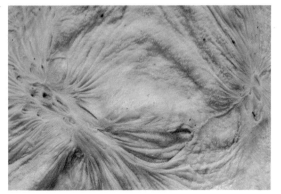

197 Scars – rumen: cattle At the surface of the rumen a few scars with a starlike appearance were seen after industrial processing. These scars are frequently due to cicatrization of necrotic lesions by *Sphaerophorus necrophorus*.

Decision: Approval with elimination of the affected tissues.

198

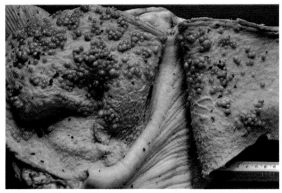

198 Papillomatosis – rumen: cattle These are small, pearly masses which have the gelatinous appearance typical of a certain type of papillomas.

Differential diagnosis: Metastasis of neoplasia; Parakeratosis.

Decision: Approval with elimination of the rumen.

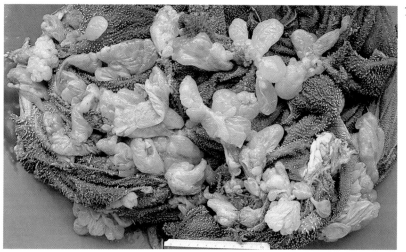

199 Mucous papillomatosis – omasum: cattle In the mucous membrane of the omasum there are numerous structures resembling common papillomas. They were papillomas developed from the squamous epithelium, with oedema of the chorion.

Decision: Approval with elimination of the omasum.

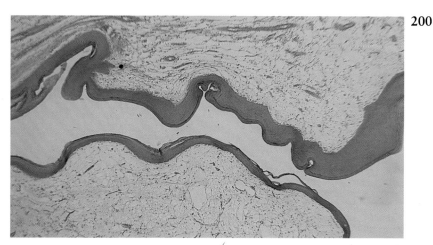

200 Mucous papillomatosis – omasum: cattle Oedema of the submucosa. The stratified epithelium has a papillomatous appearance. H. & E.

201

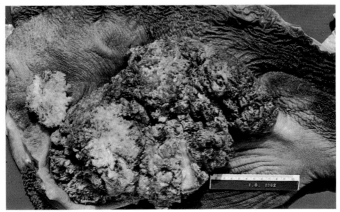

201   Squamous cell carcinoma – rumen: cattle   A voluminous cauliflower-like neoplasia in a ruminal pillar. Areas of marked congestion and an extensive attachment base, led to a diagnosis of malignant tumour, confirmed by the histopathological examination.

Differential diagnosis: Papilloma.

Decision: Total condemnation.
To perform a histopathological examination, sections should be removed from the superficial areas as well as from the base of the tumour.

202

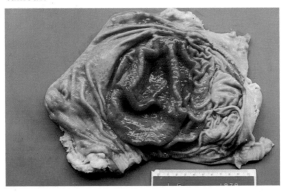

202   Haemorrhagic gastritis – stomach: swine   Acute haemorrhagic gastritis was found in the fundic region at the opening of the stomach.

Decision: Approval with elimination of the stomach.

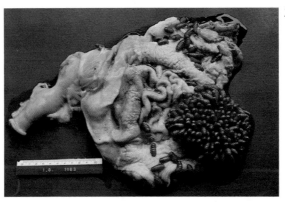

203 Gastrophilus – stomach: horse Large amounts of small brown larvae of Gastrophilus were fixed to the mucosa of the cardiac region.

Decision: Approval with elimination of the stomach.

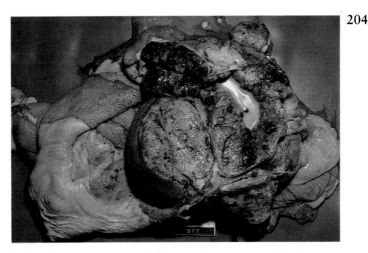

204 Leiomyoma – stomach: horse There are several globus tumours in the fundic region. They stand out from the mucosa and were composed of lardaceous yellowish tissue. One of the tumours was highly haemorrhagic. The apparent malignancy of the neoplasia was not confirmed by histopathology.

Decision: Approval with elimination of the stomach.

205

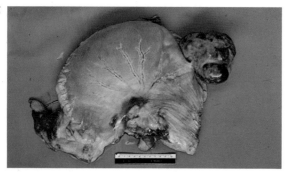

205 Leiomyosarcoma – stomach: horse A globus lobulated dark-red mass adheres by a delicate pedicle to the outside of the stomach. The histopathological examination confirmed that it was a malignant neoplasia.

Decision: Total condemnation.

206

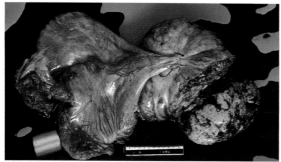

206 Leiomyosarcoma – stomach: horse A voluminous, rounded, lobulated and encapsulated neoplasia adhering to the outside of the stomach by a delicate pedicle. It was composed of lardaceous yellowish tissue with several haemorrhagic foci.

Decision: Total condemnation.

Intestine, rectum and anus

207 Rectal prolapse – intestine, anus: swine A highly haemorrhagic and oedematous mass of undetermined nature to the naked eye was microscopically identified as intestine.

Differential diagnosis: Neoplasia.

Decision: Approval with elimination of the affected tissues.

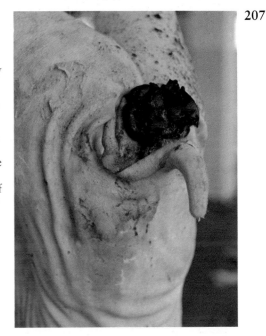

208 Intestinal tympanism: cattle The entire small intestine was dilated by an abnormal amount of gas. This phenomenon frequently occurs in cases of toxic or neural intestinal paralysis and complicated peritonitis.

Decision: Approval, if no other lesions are found, with elimination of the intestine.

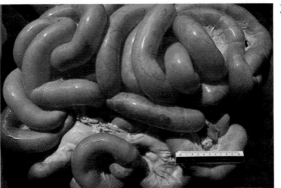

209

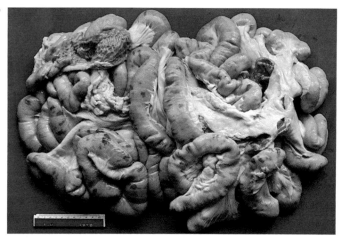

209   Focal haemorrhages – intestine: cattle   Small submucosal haemorrhages could be seen through the external layers of the intestine. They were due to traumatic damage by *Strongylus* larvae during migration.

Decision: Approval with elimination of the intestine.

210

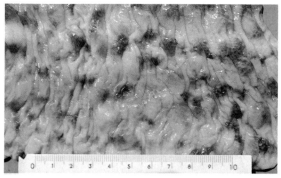

210   Focal haemorrhages – rectum: cattle   Small haemorrhages of possible parasitic origin (migrations) were located in the chorion and submucosa of the rectum.

Decision: Approval with elimination of the rectum.

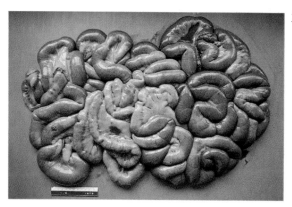

211 Haemorrhagic enteritis – intestine: cattle The small intestine was enlarged by the presence of large amounts of dark-red haemorrhagic fluid.

Differential diagnosis: Anthrax; Post-mortem hypostasis; Coccidiosis; Rinderpest; Enterotoxaemia.

Decision: Conditionally approved (heat treatment), or (alternatively) approval with elimination of the intestine depending on laboratory examination.
Laboratory examination is advisable in cases such as this.
Bacteriological examination is considered as an essential complement of direct inspection. Laboratory examinations should always be required in cases of:
(a) Emergency slaughter
(b) Presumption of contagious disease
(c) Lesions leading to a diagnosis of possible bacteraemia.
Some European countries have established that to evaluate the bacteriological contamination of the meat the laboratory has to examine the following material:
(a) *Obligatory samples:* cubic fragment of meat with 10 cm per side, aseptically collected with a myotome from the anconeus or semimembranosus muscles.
(b) *Optional samples*
(i) long bone and spleen in case of suspicion of septicaemia or disease affecting the digestive system or genital apparatus;
(ii) intact lymph node or non-punctured joint in cases of obvious or suspected lesions;
(iii) specimens of muscle or connective tissue or even of abdominal wall in order to isolate *Salmonella* in cases of suspected contamination;
(iv) samples of kidney for detection of antimicrobial products.

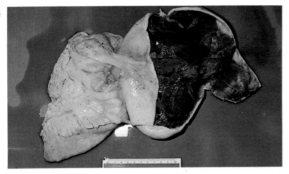

212 Encapsulated haematoma – intestine: cattle
Adherent to the large intestine by a fibrous pedicle a
large cystic-like formation was noticed. Haemorrhagic
matter showing signs of organization was found inside
the tumefaction.

Differential diagnosis: Neoplasia.

Decision: Approval with elimination of the
encapsulated haematoma.

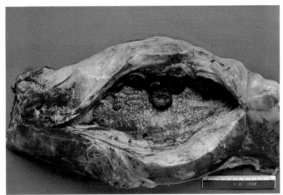

213 Non-specific rectitis – intestine: horse The wall of the rectum has
thickened due to an exudative inflammatory reaction.
The histopathological examination showed that both the chorion and the
submucosa were highly infiltrated by large amounts of fibrin. No other lesions
were found.

Differential diagnosis: Neoplasia.

Decision: Conditionally approved (heat treatment), or alternatively, approval
with elimination of the intestine, depending on laboratory examination.

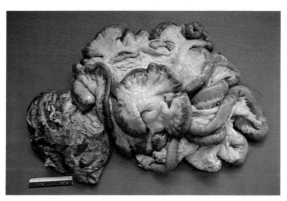

214 Acute enteritis – intestine: cattle An acute inflammatory reaction affected the intestine with predominant congestive haemorrhagic lesions. The mesenteric lymph nodes were hypertrophic and the peritoneum displayed a fibrinous inflammatory reaction.

Decision: Approval, after thermal treatment to eliminate the intestine or, alternatively, total condemnation according to results of laboratory examination.

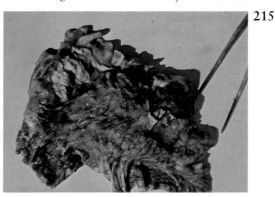

215 Button ulcers (salmonellosis) – intestine: swine Slightly prominent small ulcers with regular margins were identified in the mucosa of the caecum – the initial stage of a focal necrotic pseudomembranous enteritis which frequently occurs in cases of chronic hog cholera.

Decision: Total condemnation.

216

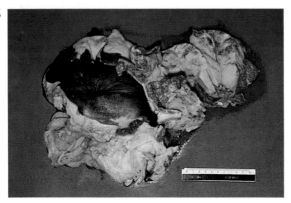

216   Perirectal inflammation – rectum: cattle   Around the end portion of the rectum a large yellow mass was found and within it small congestive areas and small necropurulent foci.

Differential diagnosis: Neoplasia.

Decision: Approval with elimination of the rectum and surrounding tissues.

217

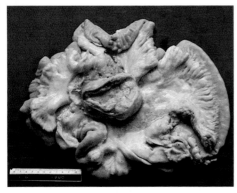

217   Tuberculosis (primary complex) – intestine and mesenteric lymph node: cattle Nodules of calcified caseous tuberculosis were identified underneath the intestinal serosa. The corresponding mesenteric lymph node was equally involved. The lesions in the lymph node justified its hypertrophy and the fluid it contained.

Differential diagnosis: Neoplasia.

Decision: Approval with elimination of the intestine.

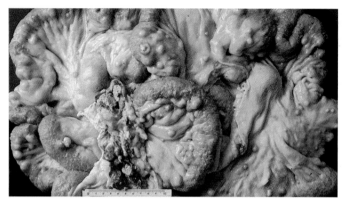

218 Calcified caseous tuberculosis – intestine: cattle Numerous prominent nodules were observed underneath the intestinal serosa. Identical structures containing necrotic yellow matter were found in the mesentery. The incision of the mesenteric lymph nodes revealed calcified caseous lesions. Some intestinal fibrinous peritonitis was clearly visible.

Differential diagnosis: Non-specific granulomas; Parasitic granulomas.

Decision: Total condemnation due to softening of the caseum.

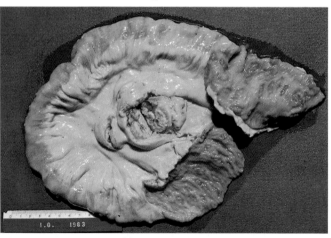

219 Ulcerative tuberculosis – intestine: cattle Numerous congestive ulcers, occasionally containing small grey tubercules, are present in the mucosa. Extensive calcified caseous lesions were found in the mesenteric lymph nodes, and similar lesions were identified in the lungs, pleura and peritoneum.

220

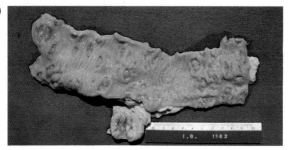

220 Ulcerative tuberculosis (detail of the previous picture) – intestine: cattle

Differential diagnosis: Necrotic-diphtheroid enteritis.

Decision: Total condemnation considering the generalisation of the tuberculosis.

221

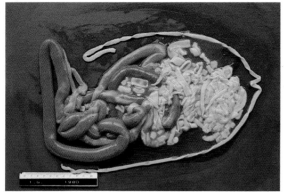

221 Parasitic enteritis (*Moniezia expansa*) – intestine: sheep Through the transparent wall of the small intestine of a young sheep, a large number of platyhelminths of the genus *Moniezia*, species *expansa*, are visible, and some fragments are outside.

Decision: Approval with elimination of the intestine.

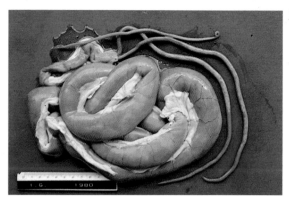

 222

222 Parasitic enteritis (*Ascaris suum*) – intestine: swine
Fragment of the intestine of a swine infected by *Ascaris suum*.

Decision: Approval with elimination of the intestine.

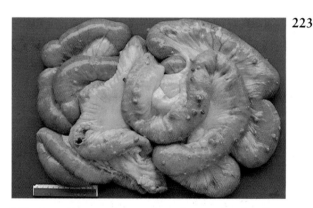 **223**

223 Parasitic granulomas – intestine: cattle Small parasitic nodules, the size of a pea could be noticed underneath the intestinal serosa. Some were yellowish and others reddish due to small haemorrhages. Where the nodules were more frequent the serosa showed a congestive inflammatory reaction.

Differential diagnosis: Nodular tuberculosis.

Decision: Approval with elimination of the intestine.

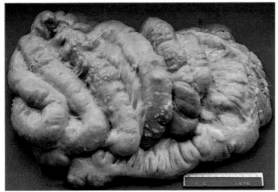

224 Parasitic granulomas – intestine: swine
Numerous prominent parasitic nodules in the colon, under the serosa, which was affected by an inflammatory reaction.

Differential diagnosis: Nodular tuberculosis.

Decision: Approval with elimination of the intestine.

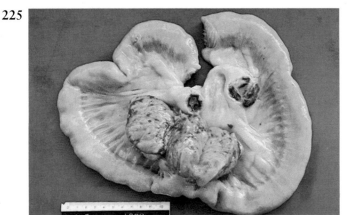

225 Leiomyoma – intestine: cattle A rounded firm encapsulated neoplasia developed from the intestinal wall. The incision showed it was formed by a yellowish tissue with dispersed small haemorrhages.

Decision: Approval with elimination of the neoplasia.

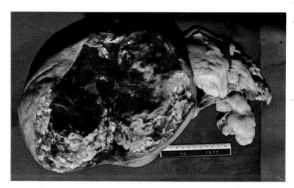

226 Fibromyoma – intestine: horse A neoplastic mass was attached to the intestinal wall by a thin pedicle. The exploratory incision showed it contained blood and fibrin and small portions of yellow lardaceous neoplastic-like tissue, all surrounded by a fibrous capsule.

Decision: Approval with elimination of the neoplasia.

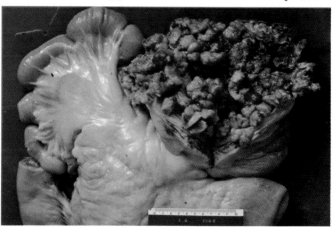

227 Adenocarcinoma – intestine: cattle A swelling of the small intestine was identified after incision as a multiple papilloma-like neoplasia. Some areas were remarkably hyperaemic and others showed signs of necrosis.

Decision: Total condemnation.

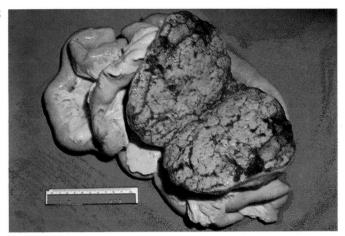

228 Leiomyosarcoma – intestine: cattle A large tumour was
attached to the intestine by a pedicle. It has a lardaceous
appearance with haemorrhagic foci.

Decision: Total condemnation.

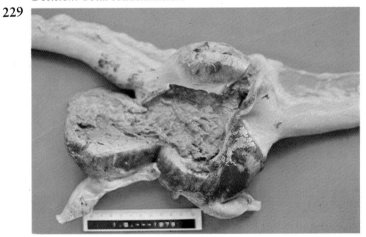

229 Malignant plasmacytoma – intestine: horse A vesicle-like
intestinal dilatation was accompanied by extensive subserosal
haemorrhages. The lumen was considerably enlarged in that area
and filled with intestinal content.

Decision: Total condemnation.

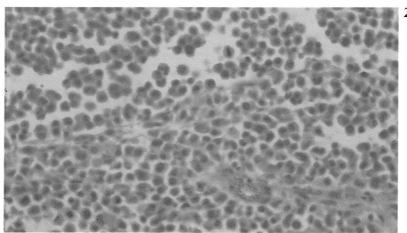

230 Malignant plasmacytoma – intestine: horse Neoplasia microscopically characterised by an abnormal proliferation of plasma cells, some of which were undergoing mitosis, indicating the growth rate of the neoplasia (plasma cells are practically the only cellular elements present in the picture). H. & E.

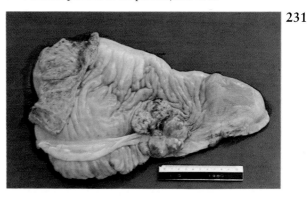

231 Undifferentiated cell sarcoma – caecum: horse Near a band of the caecum a lobulated yellow lardaceous neoplasia with focal haemorrhages was identified.

Decision: Total condemnation.

232

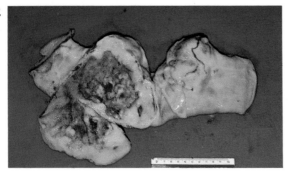

232 Undifferentiated cell sarcoma – intestine: horse
The opening of the intestine in a vesicular dilatation
showed a marked thickening of the wall, which looked
white and shiny. The mucosa was swollen, with
congestive haemorrhagic areas.

Decision: Total condemnation.

233

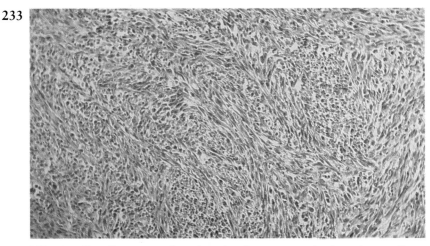

233 Spindle cell sarcoma – large intestine: horse   Strands of neoplastic cells,
oriented in different directions, a few showing signs of mitotic activity. H. & E.

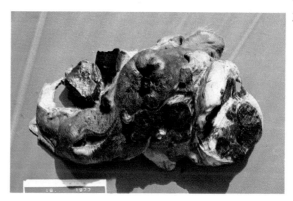

234 Melanotic sarcoma – perirectal region: horse
The tissues surrounding the final part of the rectum, the anus and the perineum showed several black and shiny neoplasias typical of melanotic neoplasia.

Decision: Total condemnation.

Liver

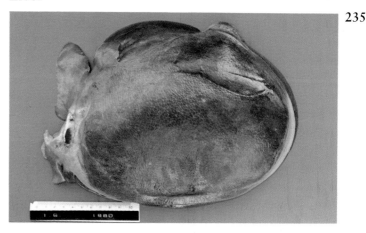

235 Congenital anomaly – liver: swine Malformation which consisted on atrophy of two lobes and compensatory hypertrophy of another. A deep fissure can be seen in the middle of the large lobe, whose perimeter is marked by fibrous tissue.

Decision: Approval with elimination of the liver.

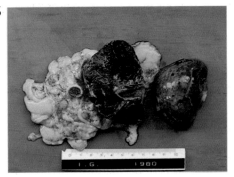

236 Accessory liver: horse Adherent to
the omentum was a reniform dark brown
body, covered by a thin capsule, which
when cut showed a liver-like structure.

Differential diagnosis: Neoplasia;
Haematoma.

Decision: Approval with elimination of the
accessory liver.

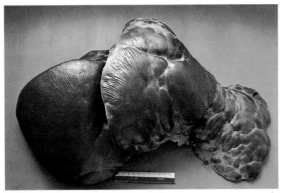

237 Supranumerary lobe and cirrhosis – liver: cattle
A large supranumerary lobe was formed from a highly
abnormal liver, which showed hyperplastic nodules
typical of cirrhosis. This demonstrates the enormous
capacity of the liver for regeneration.

Decision: Approval with elimination of the liver.

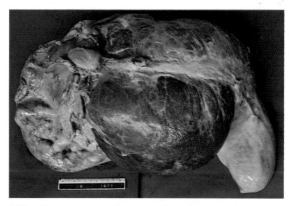

238 Compensatory hypertrophy – liver: cattle
Chronic parasitic hepatitis, with extensive destruction
of the parenchyma and compensatory hypertrophy of a
less affected area.

Differential diagnosis: Neoplasia; Haematoma.

Decision: Approval with elimination of the liver.

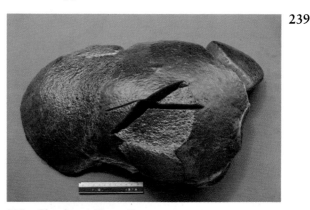

239 Cloudy swelling – liver: cattle This moderately
swollen liver showed a reddish colour and fine granular
texture, visible underneath the capsule. Palpation
showed a friable consistency.

Decision: Approval if no other lesions are found, with
elimination of the liver.

240

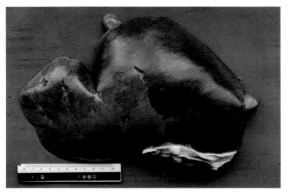

240   Localised fatty change – liver: sheep   There are two areas with distinctive coloration. The light brown area, with fat accumulation is a consequence of abnormal pulling of the hepatoligament and the vascular pedicle of the organ.

Decision: Approval with elimination of the liver.

241

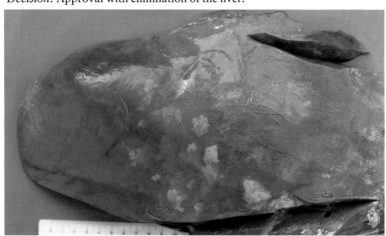

241   Focal fatty change – liver: cattle   Small, pale yellow areas are seen through the liver capsule. After incision, they had a greasy touch. Histological examination showed that these areas corresponded to focal fatty changes.

Differential diagnosis: Metastasis of neoplasia; Focal necrotic hepatitis.

Decision: Approval with elimination of the liver.

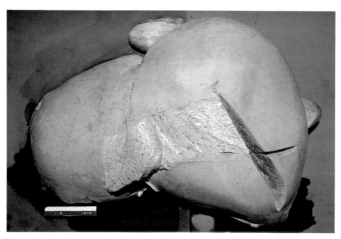

242 Fatty change – liver: cattle This highly hypertrophic yellowish organ presented a rounded profile and superficial purple lines. A considerable amount of blood drained out of the incision. The large amount of fat in the organ gave it a shiny appearance and the multiple red spots corresponded to the congested central veins. At palpation the liver was friable and it floated in water.

Differential diagnosis: Toxic fatty change due to poisoning.

Decision: Approval if no other lesions are found, with elimination of the liver.

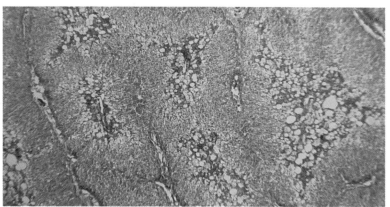

243 Fatty change – liver: cattle Congestion and steatosis of the hepatic cells in the central area of the lobules. H. & E.

244

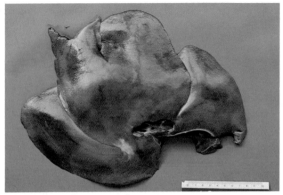

244 Fatty change – liver: swine The slightly hypertrophic organ showed a yellowish colour with demarcated red-purple areas. At palpation there was a characteristic greasy feel.

Differential diagnosis: Dietary hepatosis.

Decision: Approval with elimination of the liver.

245

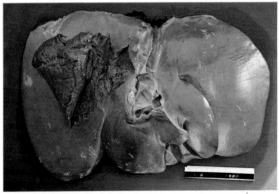

245 Fatty change – liver: horse Apart from the unusual yellowish colour the liver was particularly friable.

Differential diagnosis: Equine serum hepatitis.

Decision: Approval with elimination of the liver.

246 Hepatic dystrophy – section of liver: cattle This liver section, with thin edges well defined by connective tissue, showed softened consistency and lighter areas alternating with dark red ones.

Decision: Approval with elimination of the liver.

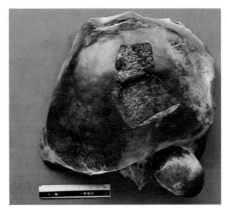

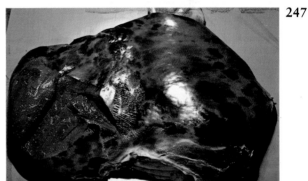

247 Melanosis (congenital) – liver: cattle At the surface and deep inside there were large black stains of variable dimensions. Their limits were not always very well defined.

Differential diagnosis: Metastasis of neoplasia; Telangiectasis; Haemosiderosis.

Decision: Approval if no other lesions are found, with elimination of the liver.

248

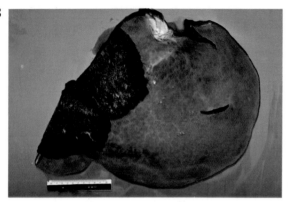

248 Passive congestion – section of liver: cattle The abnormal dark colour was due to serious stasis related to endocarditis in the tricuspid valve.

Decision: Total condemnation due to the endocarditis.

249

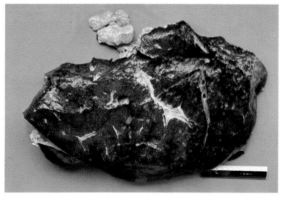

249 Congestive haemorrhagic inflammation – section of liver: cattle This dark red section of liver showed extensive haemorrhagic areas and numerous irregular dry necrotic foci. The hilum lymph nodes were moist and shiny, suggesting the existence of an inflammatory reaction.

Differential diagnosis: Venous hyperaemia (cardiopathy).

Decision: Approval, if no other lesions are found, with elimination of the liver.

250 Congestive sclerosis – liver: swine The liver showed clear modifications of its colour and considerable increase in thickness. The fine granular surface, due to sclerosis of circulatory origin, produced a sandpaper effect at palpation.

Differential diagnosis: Fatty change; Dietary hepatitis.

Decision: Approval with elimination of the liver.

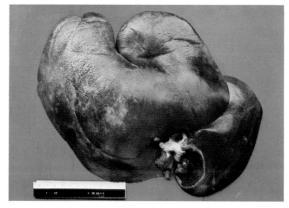

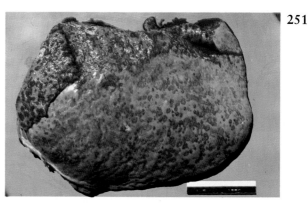

251 Telangiectasis – section of liver: cattle The surface of the liver was highly irregular due to multiple small purple depressive areas. The same change was noticed deep within the organ.

Differential diagnosis: Melanosis; Metastasis of neoplasia; Localized haemosiderosis.

Decision: Approval with elimination of the liver.

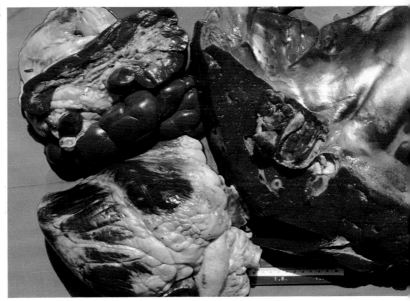

252 General systemic reaction – viscera: cattle The organs shown in the picture were highly congested and the heart showed some blue-purple patches. The lymph nodes were swollen and congested.

Decision: Total condemnation.

Note: Apart from the changes in the organs shown in the picture, the carcase presented signs of jaundice and the perirenal tissues showed extensive haemorrhages. The enquiry which took place after the post-mortem inspection revealed that the consignment of animals presenting the above described lesions had been simultaneously inoculated with two vaccines 14 days before slaughter. In cases of general systemic reaction several authors consider the following fundamental factors that have to be noted at the post-mortem inspection:
(a) insufficient bleeding; (b) subcutaneous fat changes; (c) serosal changes;
(d) peculiar serosal smells; (e) joint changes; (f) lymph node changes;
(g) musculature changes; (h) diffuse parenchymal changes.

253 Telangiectasis and fibrosis – liver: cattle
The progressive compression of the hepatic trabeculae led to degenerative and necrotic changes of the hepatic cells, which were finally replaced by fibrous tissue. H. & E.

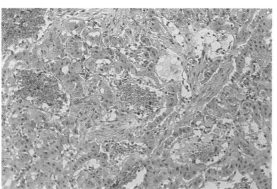

253

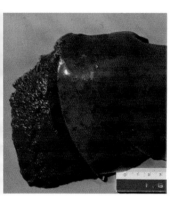

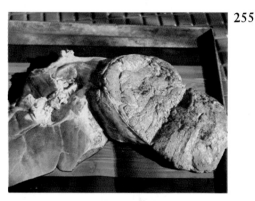

255

254 Subcapsular haemorrhages (echymosis) – section of liver: cattle
Numerous small dark stains were identified underneath the capsule, corresponding to small haemorrhages of unidentified origin.

Differential diagnosis: Melanosis; Metastasis of neoplasia; Haemosiderosis.

Decision: Approval with elimination of the liver.

255 Haematoma – liver: cattle   A considerable haematoma, possibly of traumatic origin, was surrounded by a fibrous capsule and attached to the liver by a large pedicle. The yellow colour was due to the presence of haemoglobin-derived pigments.

Differential diagnosis: Neoplasia.

Decision: Approval with elimination of the haematoma.

256

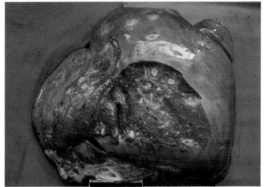

256 Focal necrotic hepatitis – liver: cattle
The liver parenchyma was seeded at the surface and deep inside with yellow polycyclic nodules (1–2 cm in diameter) surrounded by a congestive halo.

Differential diagnosis: Necrobacillosis; Tuberculosis; Metastasis of neoplasia.

Decision: Approval with elimination of the liver or, alternatively, conditioned (heat treatment), according to results of laboratory examination.

257

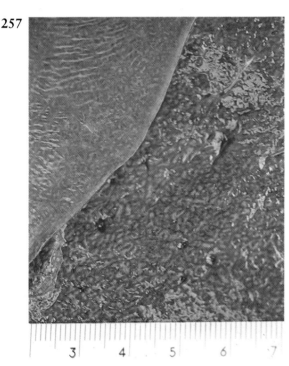

257 Focal necrotic hepatitis – section of liver: cattle Multiple yellow foci can be clearly seen under the liver capsule, contrasting with the normal parenchyma, which corresponded to areas of necrosis.

Decision: Approval for consumption is conditioned to thermal treatment, with elimination of the liver, pending the results of laboratory examination.

258 Perilobular icterogenic hepatitis – liver: horse The liver was enlarged, with round edges, and was bronze-green due to retention of biliary pigments subsequent to perilobular sclerosis. It was also abnormally divided.

Decision: Approval with elimination of the liver.

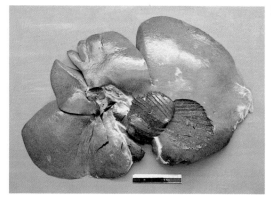

258

259 Hepatic abscess – liver (carcase) : cattle During evisceration an opening of an abscess occurred. It was located in the liver but in close relation to the right kidney. Its localisation may erroneously suggest a purulent nephritis which has different inspection criteria.

Decision: Approval if no other lesions are found, with elimination of the affected tissues.

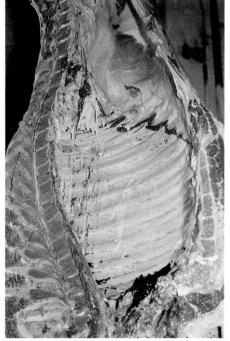

259

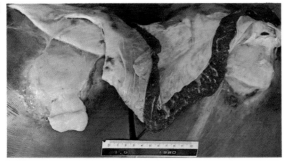

260 Hepatic abscesses – liver: cattle In the cranial face of the liver, adherent to the diaphragm, two abscesses (approximately 5 cm in diameter) were seen, surrounded by a chronic inflammatory reaction. The accidental opening of one of them showed a pasty yellow-green pus.

Differential diagnosis: Tuberculosis; Actinobacillosis.

Decision: Approval with elimination of the liver and diaphragm.

 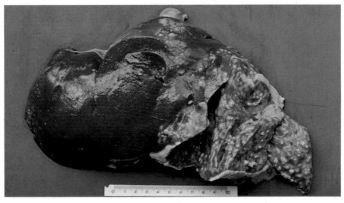

261 Hepatic abscesses – liver: sheep The right side of the liver showed numerous small abscesses containing a yellow lumpy pus and surrounded by fibrous tissue.

Decision: Approval if no other lesions are found, with elimination of the liver or conditioned approved (heat treatment), according to results of laboratory examination.

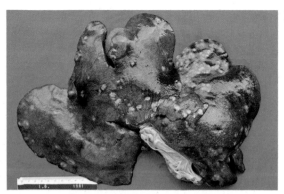

262 Hepatic abscesses – liver: swine Large numbers of small well-defined greenish nodules were found in a liver with fatty change. Some of these nodules showed a calcified core.

Decision: Approval, if no other lesions are found, with elimination of the liver.

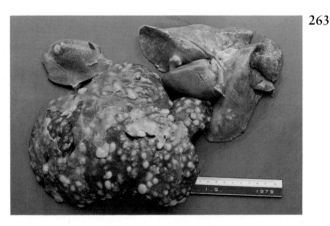

263 Pyohaemic abscesses – viscera: sheep A profusion of small abscesses, containing yellow thick pus were seen in the liver. Identical lesions were present in the spleen and lungs suggesting septicaemia.

Differential diagnosis: Hydatidosis.

Decision: Total condemnation.

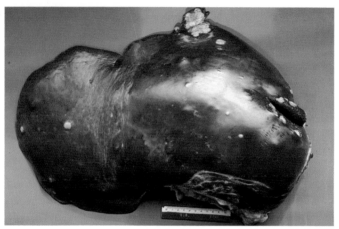

264 Non-specific granulomas – liver: cattle Yellow nodules of different sizes seen at variable depth at the surface of the liver. The nodules were not separated from the parenchyma by any particular reaction. The hepatic lymph nodes were not reactive.

Differential diagnosis: Metastasis of neoplasia; Tuberculosis; Necrobacillosis; Actinobacillosis or actinomycosis.

Decision: Approval with elimination of the liver.

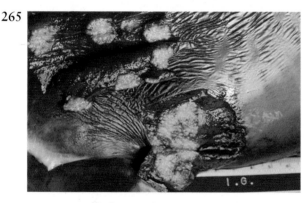

265 Non-specific granulomas – liver: cattle
Magnification of the lesions shown in **264**.

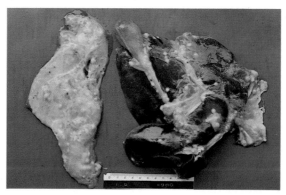

266 Non-specific granulomas – section of liver and peritoneum: sheep Small yellowish nodules were identified at the surface and inside the liver and in the peritoneum. They had the microscopical structure of granulomas of unknown aetiology. Generalised process.

Differential diagnosis: Tuberculosis; Abscesses.

Decision: Total condemnation.

267 Non-specific granulomas – liver and spleen: swine Yellow lardaceous nodules of very different sizes in the liver, some of them slightly prominent under the capsule. Identical nodules also present in the spleen, one of which resembled a tumour.

Differential diagnosis: Metastasis of neoplasia; Tuberculosis.

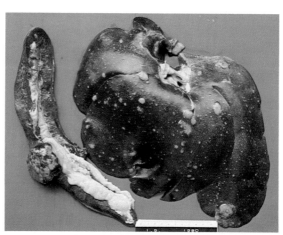

Decision: Approval, with elimination of the liver and spleen, subject to laboratory examination.

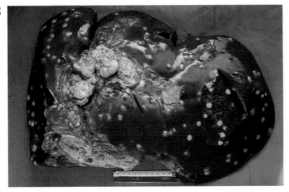

268 Tuberculosis (slow generalisation) – liver: cattle
Large numbers of caseocalcified nodules of identical size
suggest a sudden haematogeneity. The lymph nodes of
the hilum showed identical caseocalcified nodules,
apparently at the same stage of evolution. The lungs and
pleura were also affected in the same way.

Differential diagnosis: Pyogenic abscesses;
Necrobacillosis; Metastasis of neoplasia;
Actinobacillosis.

Decision: Total condemnation.

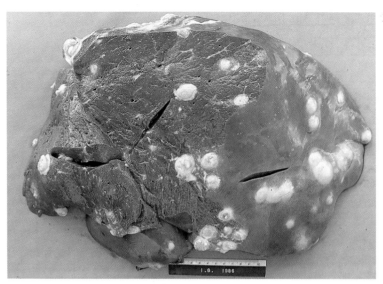

269 Actinobacillosis – liver: cattle   Under the capsule there are numerous greenish-yellow nodules. When these were sectioned a yellow elastic pus could be seen in the central core. Peripherally they were surrounded by fibrous tissue which compressed the nodules, making them prominent at the incision.

Differential diagnosis: Tuberculosis; Non-specific granulomas; Focal hepatitis; Parasitic granulomas; Metastasis of neoplasias.

Decision: Approval with elimination of the organ.

270

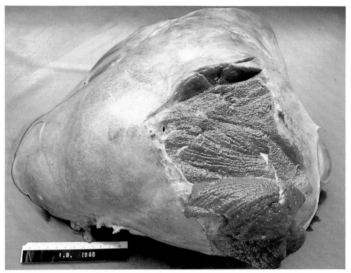

270 Fibrosis – liver: cattle Progressive fibrosis of the liver, involving the capsule, which was considerably thickened, and the parenchyma. The organ was atrophic, and of considerably hard consistency. At microscopic examination initial lesions of cirrhosis were identified.

Decision: Approval with elimination of the liver.

271

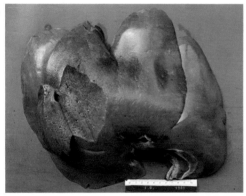

271 Chronic interstitial hepatitis – liver: swine The liver was of normal size, but of hard consistency, and in the overall light-brown colour some purple stains were seen, together with numerous small superficial depressions. Where the organ was cut the augmented consistency was seen distinctively.

Differential diagnosis: Fatty change.

Decision: Approval with elimination of the liver.

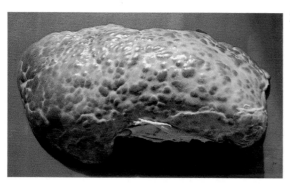

272 Atrophic cirrhosis – liver: cattle The profile is considerably changed due to the multiple light-brown nodules, prominent under the capsule. In between the nodules large amounts of fibrous tissue, infiltrated by biliary pigments, give it a yellow colour.

Decision: Approval with elimination of the liver.

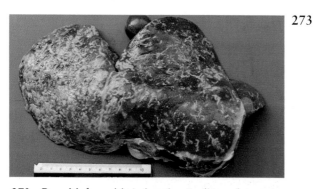

273 Parasitic hepatitis (migrations) – liver: sheep
The liver was highly modified due to a high number of lesions caused by the passage of parasites. The straw-coloured lesions are the remains of destroyed hepatic cells mixed with polymorphonucleated cells – neutrophils and eosinophils.

Decision: Approval with elimination of the liver.

274

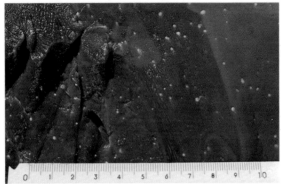

274 Disseminated calcified parasitic nodules – section of liver: horse Many small rounded white nodules were present in the parenchyma. These nodules were difficult to cut due to calcification of the necrotic foci made by migrating strongyle larvae.

Differential diagnosis: Tuberculosis; Non-specific granulomas.

Decision: Approval with elimination of the liver.

275

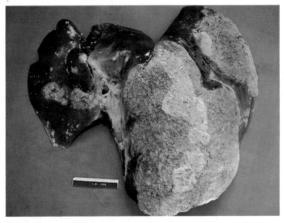

275 Disseminated calcified parasitic nodules – liver: horse The surface of the right lobe was deeply modified. A large number of small nodules with dystrophic calcification were formed by migrating strongyle larvae.

Differential diagnosis: Tuberculosis.

Decision: Approval with elimination of the liver.

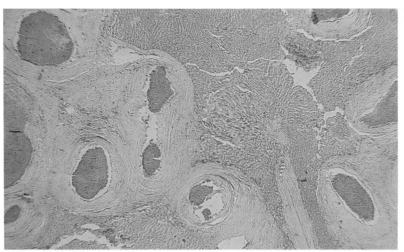

276   Disseminated calcified parasitic nodules – liver: horse   Numerous calcified foci surrounded by fibrous tissue can be seen.
H. & E. after decalcification in acidulated solution.

277   Parasitic hepatitis – liver: swine   Numerous milk spots due to migrating larvae of *Ascaris* were seen at the surface of the liver, underneath the capsule.

Differential diagnosis: Tuberculosis (avian type).

Decision: Approval with elimination of the liver.

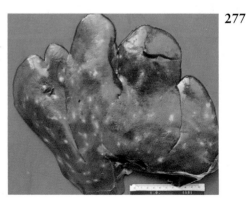

278

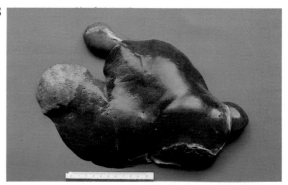

278   Parasitic hepatitis – liver: sheep   Part of the left lobe is yellowish-green with the lobular structure particularly well-defined. The limits of the affected area are very sharp and the incision shows a deep infection by *Fasciola hepatica* trematodes that have completely blocked the biliary ducts.

Decision: Approval with elimination of the liver.

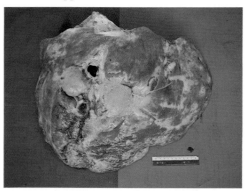

279   Parasitic hepatitis – section of liver: cattle   White irregular cords are visible, slightly prominent under the capsule, corresponding to biliary ducts affected by a chronic inflammatory reaction due to the irritant action of the *Fasciola hepatica* trematodes.

Decision: Approval with elimination of the liver.

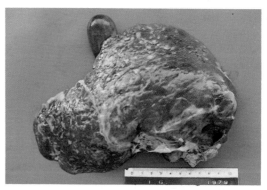

280   **Parasitic hepatitis: sheep**   The markedly
atrophic liver clearly shows an irregular surface
due to cicatricial retraction and the thickening of
the capsule, sometimes assuming a nodular
feature or appearing as streaks a few centimetres
long.

Decision: Approval with elimination of the liver.

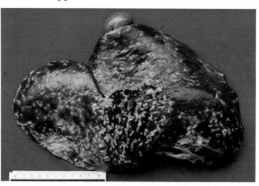

281   **Parasitic hepatitis (dicrocoeliasis) – liver:
sheep**   Small nodules and yellow irregular
streaks were noticed by the external observation.
Inside, many biliary ducts were enlarged and had
thickened walls as a consequence of *Dicrocoelium*
infection.

Decision: Approval with elimination of the liver.

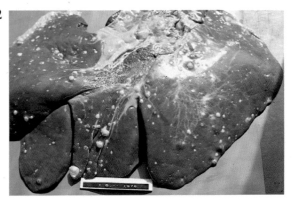

282 Parasitic hepatitis (hydatidosis) – liver: horse
The liver was seeded with small prominent vesicles
containing a transparent fluid, with the typical
appearance of hydatid cysts. It should be noted that
these vesicles assume in horses a remarkably reduced
size in comparison with the hydatid cysts found in other
slaughtered animals.

Decision: Approval with elimination of the liver.

283

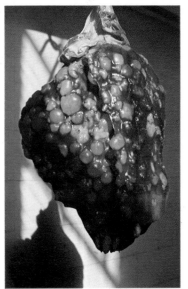

**283 Parasitic hepatitis (hydatidosis) –
liver: swine** The liver was deeply modified
due to large numbers of hydatid cysts which
had replaced most of the parenchyma.

Decision: Approval with elimination of the
liver.

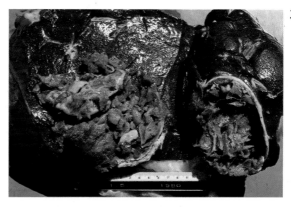

284 Parasitic hepatitis (hydatid cyst) – section of liver: cattle Incision into a tumour revealed an altered hydatid cyst with marked sclerosis of its capsule. The cavity was filled with membranes infiltrated by biliary pigments.

Decision: Approval with elimination of the hepatic lesion.

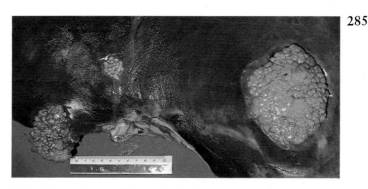

285 Polycystic or multivesicular hydatidosis – section of liver: cattle At the surface of the liver masses of variable diameter were noticed, made of aggregates of small vesicles the size of a pea, which contained a small amount of transparent fluid together with solidified material.

Differential diagnosis: Tuberculosis; Actinobacillosis or actinomycosis.

Decision: Approval with elimination of the liver.

286

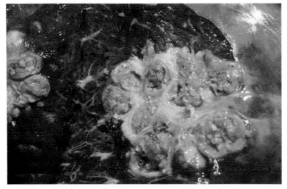

286 Polycystic or multivesicular hydatidosis: cattle
Close-up of a section of one of the vesicular aggregates
shown in **285**. The vesicles contained a yellow solidified
material and were surrounded by fibrous tissue.

287

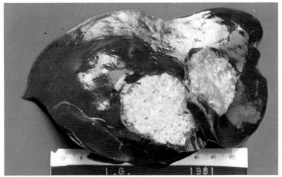

**287 Polycystic or multivesicular hydatidosis – section
of liver: sheep**   An aggregate of small vesicles was
found at the surface of the liver. Fibrous tissue isolated
each of these vesicles as can be seen in the picture
shown.

Decision: Approval with elimination of the liver.

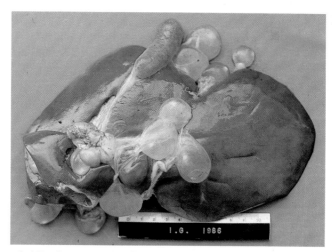

288 Cysticercosis (*Cysticercus tenuicollis*) – liver: sheep Numerous vesicles, containing a translucent fluid were found in the surface of the liver, attached to the capsule by a thin pedicle. Inside some of the vesicles a scolex of *Cysticercus tenuicollis* could be seen.

Differential diagnosis: Hydatidosis.

Decision: Approval with elimination of the organ.

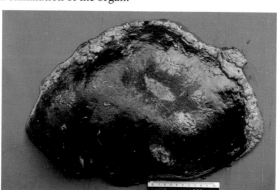

289 Granulomatous parasitic perihepatitis – section of liver: horse The border of the liver shows marked sclerosis of the capsule, with large amounts of small nodules at that site. The sectioned nodules contain pus, surrounded by a solid slightly greenish tissue. Calcified parasitic nodules were also noticed in the parenchyma.

Decision: Approval with elimination of the liver.

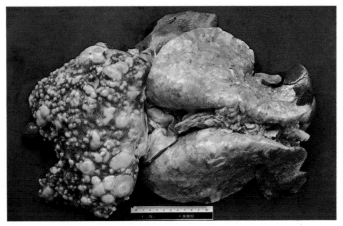

290 Unilocular hydatidosis – viscera: sheep Many hydatid cysts were seen in the liver. However, the fact that some showed small vesicles together with larger ones suggested that a secondary hydatidosis had occurred. Hydatid cysts were also present in the lungs.

Decision: Approval with elimination of the liver.

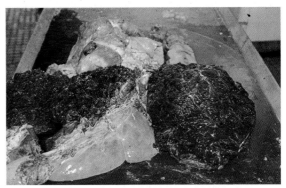

291 Haemangioma – liver: cattle A large globular soft swelling at the back of the liver. A considerable amount of blood drained out of the incision. The cut surface had some resemblance to lungs affected by bronchopneumonia.

Differential diagnosis: Haematoma.

Decision: Approval with elimination of the liver.

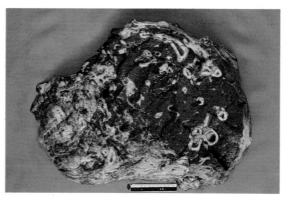

292   Malignant evolution (adenocarcinoma) of parasitic hepatitis – section of liver: cattle   Marked hyperplastic and sclerosing reaction of the biliary ducts due to severe infection by trematodes. Apart from chronic parasitic cholangitis, the parenchyma on the left side of the picture showed initial neoplastic lesions corresponding to an adenocarcinoma.

Decision: Total condemnation.

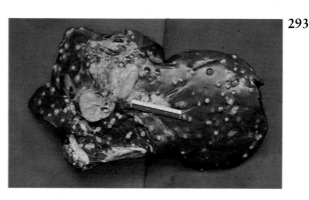

293   Hepatocellular carcinoma – liver: cattle   The parenchyma was invaded by small yellow nodules with round profile. Many of these, composed of necrotic matter surrounded by fibrous tissue, were parasitic nodules. The less well defined ones, which were vascularized, shiny and lardaceous, were neoplastic.

Differential diagnosis: Necrobacillosis; Tuberculosis; Actinobacillosis or actinomycosis.

Decision: Total condemnation.

294

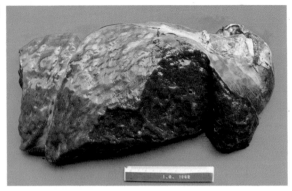

294 Hepatocellular carcinoma – section of liver: cattle
Some aspects resemble telangiectasis. However, the
marked hyperaemia, absence of tissue loss and the
identification of small areas of newly formed lighter
tissue suggested a neoplastic process.

Differential diagnosis: Telangiectasis.

Decision: Total condemnation.

295

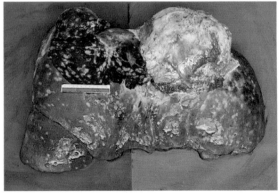

295 Hepatocellular carcinoma: cattle A very large
abscess was located in the left lobe of the liver and most
of the parenchyma was invaded by shiny yellow masses
of irregular profile and hard consistency, which were
diagnosed as malignant neoplasia.

Differential diagnosis: Necrobacillosis; Necrotic focal
hepatitis.

Decision: Total condemnation.

296 Hepatocellular carcinoma – section of liver: cattle A tumoral pearly like tissue proliferated and destroyed the liver. Only a few isolated areas of tissue remained. A heavy infection by *Fasciola hepatica* was also taking place.

Differential diagnosis: Atrophic cirrhosis.

Decision: Total condemnation.

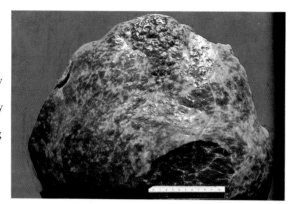

296

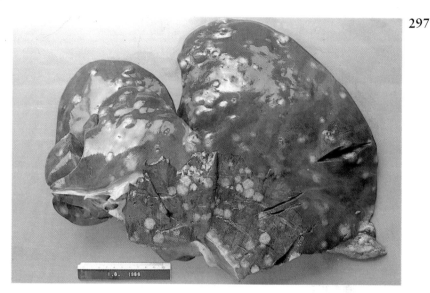

297

297 Hepatocellular carcinoma – section of liver: horse Small yellow nodules of more or less regular profile and 1 cm in diameter, were dispersed in the parenchyma, corresponding to a primary generalization of a hepatocellular carcinoma of trabecular type.

Differential diagnosis: Focal necrotic hepatitis; Necrobacillosis; Unspecific granulomas.

Decision: Total condemnation.

298

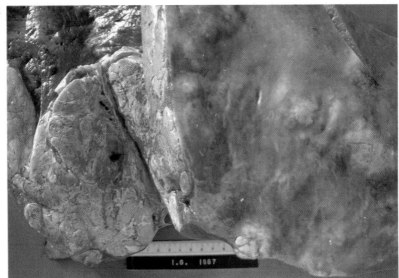

298 Hepatocellular carcinoma – section of liver: cattle The liver showed a neoplasia consisting of white or yellowish-white nodules of irregular profile, slightly prominent under the capsule or deeply buried in the parenchyma.

Decision: Total condemnation.

299

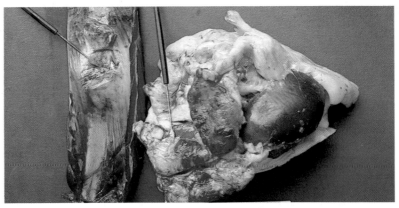

299 Metastasis of hepatocellular carcinoma – adrenal gland and rib: horse The adrenal gland and one rib showed neoplastic nodules due to secondary generalization of the neoplasia.

Decision: Total condemnation.

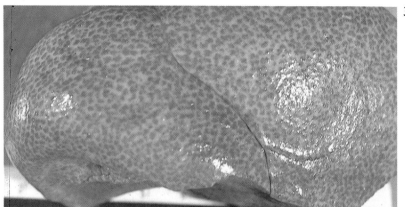

300 Carcinoma – liver: cattle The liver was pale due to large amounts of lardaceous tissue, which assumed a reticular arrangement, marking the lobular structure of the organ.

Decision: Total condemnation.

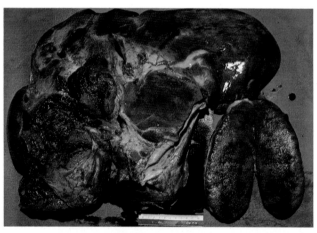

301 Carcinoma – liver – sarcoma – superficial cervical lymph node: cattle
Two different neoplasias developed in the same animal. The liver, which showed clear signs of parasitic cholangitis on the right side, had a malignant tumour at its left. The neoplastic tissue was greenish, shiny and lardaceous. The considerably enlarged lymph node displayed haemorrhages in the medulla and the cortex was invaded by a clearly neoplastic tissue.

Decision: Total condemnation.

302

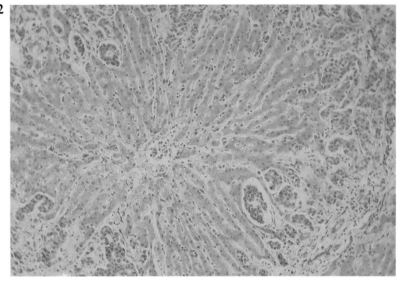

302 **Metastasis of a bronchial carcinoma – liver: horse**   The liver was affected by the secondary dissemination of a carcinoma originated in the bronchi. H. & E.

303

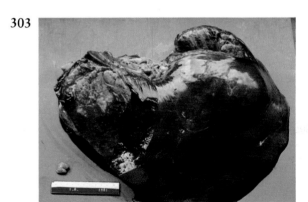

303 **Malignant trabecular hepatoma – liver: cattle**
The two rounded swellings at the surface are paler than the normal tissue. They were formed of a yellowish neoplastic tissue, showing multiple haemorrhages.

Decision: Total condemnation.

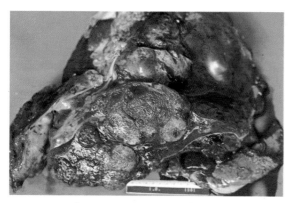

304   Malignant trabecular hepatoma – section of liver: cattle   There are several pale prominent swellings at the surface of the liver, and also within the organ. They were made of yellowish lardaceous tissue with focal haemorrhages.

Decision: Total condemnation.

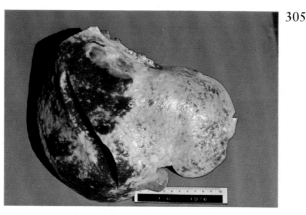

305   Adenocarcinoma – liver: sheep   The whole left lobe was replaced by a yellowish shiny tissue, slightly more consistent than the liver itself. The right lobe was invaded by small nodules of the same tissue.

Decision: Total condemnation.

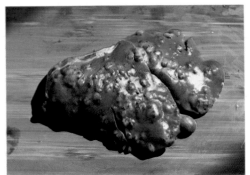

306 Adenocarcinoma – liver: sheep Several clear nodules of different size invaded the liver. Some showed a central umbilicated depression suggesting their malignant nature.

Decision: Total condemnation.

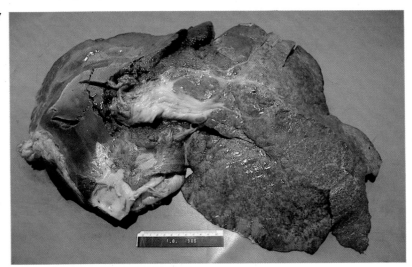

307 Metastasis from mesothelioma – liver: horse The liver, with a softened consistency, was invaded by the metastasis of a mesothelioma located near the stomach. The small metastatic nodules were deforming the surface of the liver, appearing as fine granules under the capsule.

Differential diagnosis: Tuberculosis; Calcified parasitic nodules.

Decision: Total condemnation.

308 Spindle-cell sarcoma – liver: horse Yellow neoplasias of different sizes are present in the liver. The cut surface had a characteristic shine. The parenchyma around the larger tumours was markedly green due to the compression of the tumours over the biliary ducts.

Decision: Total condemnation.

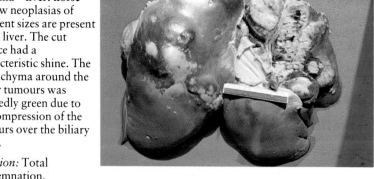

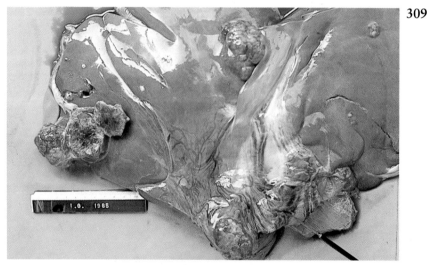

309 Undifferentiated cell sarcoma – section of the liver: horse There are prominent tumoral nodules under the capsule, of lardaceous appearance, with haemorrhagic centre and firm consistency. One of the nodules was highly irrigated by dilated, seemingly varicose blood vessels.

Differential diagnosis: Non-specific granulomas; Actinobacillosis or actinomycosis.

Decision: Total condemnation.

310

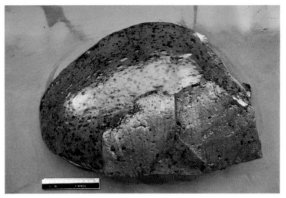

**310 Metastasis of undifferentiated cell sarcoma –
section of liver: horse** The liver is invaded by small
dark nodules, slightly prominent under the capsule.

Differential diagnosis: Melanosis; Telangiectasis;
Subcapsular haemorrhages.

Decision: Total condemnation.

311

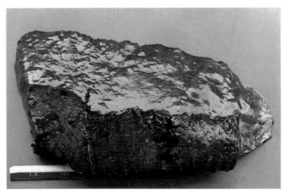

**311 Metastasis of undifferentiated cell sarcoma –
section of liver: horse** This highly irregular light-
brown liver is deeply invaded by secondary tumoral
nodules, some of which are haemorrhagic. These
nodules were metastases of a sarcoma located in the
spleen.

Decision: Total condemnation.

312 Metastasis of undifferentiated cell sarcoma of the spleen – liver: horse The trabecular structure was interrupted in some areas by the metastasis of a sarcoma located in the spleen. The lacunal irrigation, typical of sarcomas can be clearly seen. H. & E.

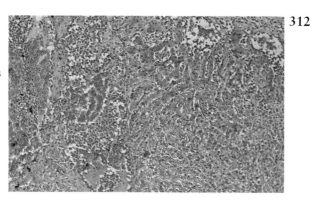

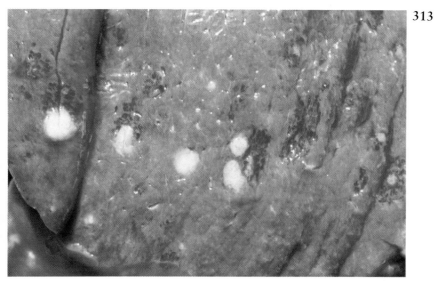

313 Metastasis of undifferentiated cell sarcoma – liver: horse The exploratory incision of a splenic tumour revealed the existence of numerous rounded yellow nodules due to metastatic diffusion. The growth of the secondary tumours originated local circulatory disturbances which assumed a feature similar to telangiectasis.

Differential diagnosis: Focal necrotic hepatitis.

Decision: Total condemnation.

314

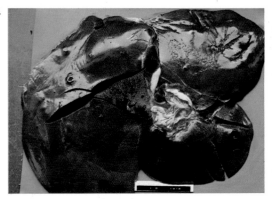

314   Metastasis of melanotic neoplasia – liver: horse   Round prominent black nodules of regular profile were identified at the surface of the liver. Some of them were umbilicated. Identical nodules were seen within the organ.

Differential diagnosis: Haematomas.

Decision: Total condemnation.

315

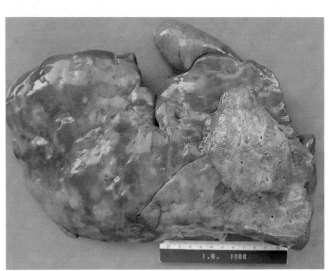

315   Lymphoblastic lymphosarcoma – liver: sheep
Discoloration of the liver was evident, through the appearance of clear areas at the surface and within the organ. Histological examination showed the accumulation of lymphoblasts in clear areas, some of which were undergoing mitotic division. These cells were compressing the liver cell cords and destroying the hepatic cells.

Differential diagnosis: Steatosis (fatty change); Hepatitis.

Decision: Total condemnation.

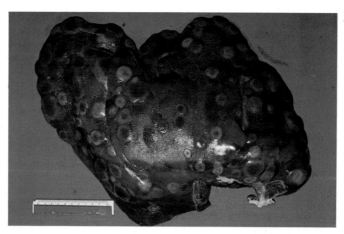

316 Lymphoblastic leukosis – liver: swine Numerous round and regular nodules in the parenchyma, the superficial ones being slightly prominent. They are lardaceous, shiny and pinkish, reddened in the centre due to haemorrhages.

Decision: Total condemnation.

Biliary tract (gall bladder)

317

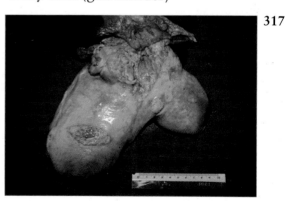

317 Bifid gall bladder: cattle Development disturbances not uncommon in cattle and without significance in the meat quality.

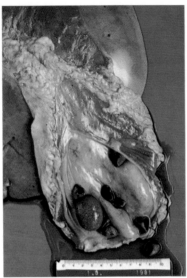

318 Calculi – gall bladder: cattle Nine biliary calculi were found inside the gall bladder, eight of the same morphological type and a ninth ovoid-shaped. The last one was fixed inside the bile duct (ductus choledochus).

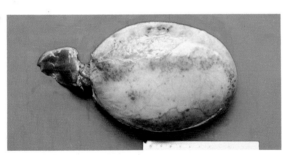

319 Petechial haemorrhages – gall bladder: cattle
The slightly oedematous wall of the gall bladder showed congested vessels and petechial haemorrhages.

Decision: Approval with elimination of the gall bladder.
Note: The petechial haemorrhages may be part of a more general pathological situation with repercussion in the meat quality. In such cases the decision will be made accordingly.

320 Acute cholecystitis – gall bladder: cattle A congestive haemorrhagic inflammatory reaction affecting the gall bladder, whose walls were thickened due to an inflammatory oedema.

Decision: Approval with elimination of the gall bladder.

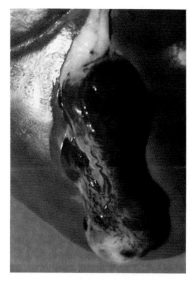

321 Acute cholecystitis – gall bladder: cattle An acute inflammatory reaction in the gall bladder caused by congestion, oedema and petechial haemorrhages.

Decision: Approval with elimination of the gall bladder.

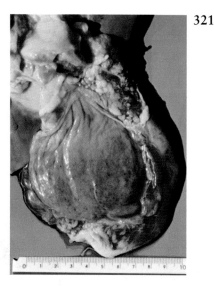

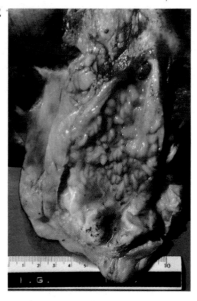

322 Polypoid cholecystitis: cattle
Numerous polyps of the mucosa are apparent, possibly resulting from a chronic inflammatory reaction.

Differential diagnosis: Neoplasia.

Decision: Approval with elimination of the gall bladder.

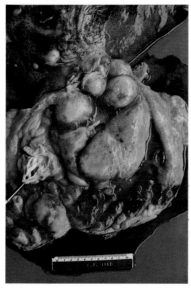

323 Hydatid cyst – liver and gall bladder: cattle The serosa of the gall bladder was congested and palpation showed several spherical masses of various sizes. In the wall which was sectioned numerous vesicles are visible, containing a limpid fluid like water. Identical vesicles were seen in the liver near the gall bladder.

Decision: Approval with elimination of the liver.

324 Proliferative adenomatosis with signs of malignancy – gall bladder: cattle Observation and palpation revealed a considerable thickening of the gall bladder wall. This was due to proliferation of the mucosa which was roughly plicated.

Differential diagnosis: Cholecystitis.

Decision: Total condemnation.

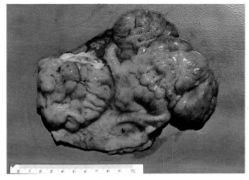

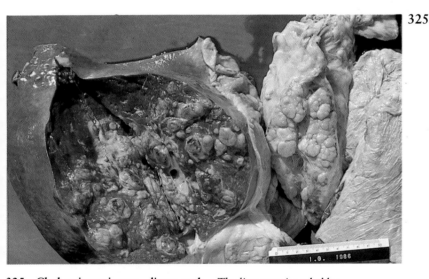

325 Cholangiocarcinoma – liver: cattle The liver was invaded by multinodular circular masses, bulging at the cut surface, sometimes depressed in the centre. Their diameter varied from a few millimetres to approximately 4 cm. In some areas these nodules were similar to lesions of parasitic cholangitis and in other areas they resembled a secondary tumour. The mediastinal lymph node was highly invaded by metastatic dissemination.

Decision: Total condemnation.

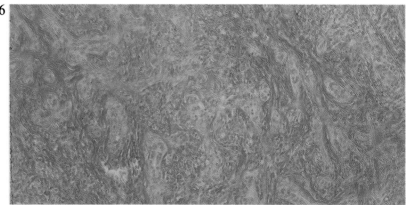

326 Cholangiocarcinoma – liver: cattle A neoplasia of the biliary ducts determined considerable destruction of the liver parenchyma. The neoplastic biliary ducts are surrounded by a stroma rich in collagen, which seems to oppose the tumour growth. Van Gieson.

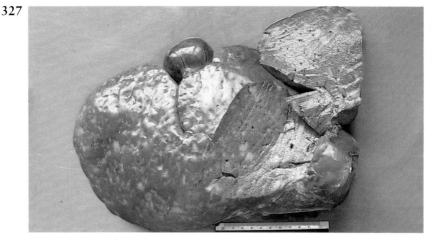

327 Cholangiocarcinoma – liver: sheep The liver, which was abnormally discoloured, had a very irregular surface due to the existence of multiple depressions in the light-coloured areas. The incision of the organ showed several pale rounded nodules within the parenchyma.

Differential diagnosis: Focal hepatitis.

Decision: Total condemnation.

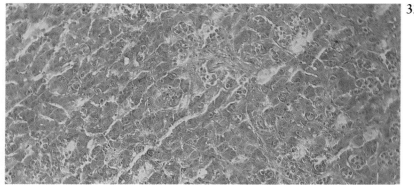

328 Cholangiocarcinoma – liver: sheep The neoplasia, at an initial stage of development, had an abnormal cellular growth which interrupted here and there the normal trabecular architecture of the organ, assuming the typical morphology of biliary ducts. H. & E.

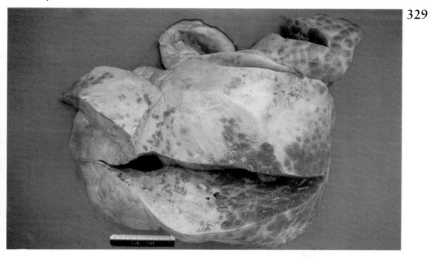

329 Cholangiocarcinoma – liver: cattle The organ presented deep colour changes and surface irregularities, which, particularly in some areas, assumed the morphology of atrophic cirrhosis. The consistency of the organ was deeply increased, the liver difficult to cut.

Differential diagnosis: Atrophic cirrhosis.

Decision: Total condemnation.

330

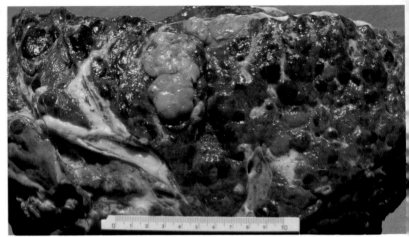

330 Cholangiocarcinoma – liver: cattle The incision of a highly irregular liver, revealed the multifocal development of neoplastic tissue. Small dark nodules bulged above the cut surface. In the areas of more advanced evolution the neoplastic tissue was pinkish-white.

Decision: Total condemnation.

331

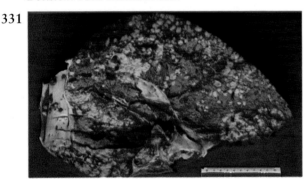

331 Cholangiocarcinoma – section of liver: cattle
The surface of the liver showed yellow subcapsular stains. The section revealed the presence of numerous yellow nodules, sometimes confluent, which seemed to arise from the biliary ducts.

Differential diagnosis: Tuberculosis; Actinobacillosis; Necrobacillosis; Non-specific granulomas.

Decision: Total condemnation.

Pancreas

332 Calculi (lithiasis) – pancreas: cattle When the pancreas was manipulated during evisceration the presence of small hard round bodies was clearly felt. The incision of the pancreatic duct revealed the presence of small white calculi all of identical size.

Decision: Approval with elimination of the pancreas.

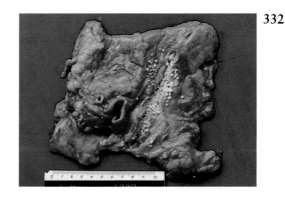

332

333 Abscess – pancreas: cattle There is a localised increase in the thickness of the organ, with an ovoid shape. Each contains pus, more or less solidified, surrounded by a fibrous capsule.

Decision: Approval with elimination of the pancreas.

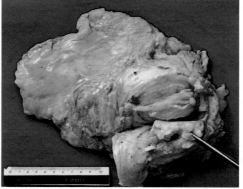

333

334

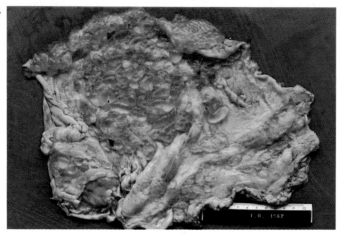

334 Lymphatic cysts – peritoneum: cattle The lymphatics, which usually cannot be seen, were transformed into a multitude of elongated vesicles containing a transparent fluid. This is probably a congenital malformation.

Decision: Approval with elimination of the affected areas.

335

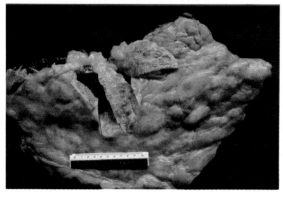

335 Necrosis of the subperitoneal fat: cattle The abnormally thickened subperitoneal fat was affected by massive fat necrosis.

Decision: Approval with elimination of the affected fat.

336 Abscess – peritoneum: cattle
A very large abscess was located near the diaphragm, compressing it near the sternum. It contained large amounts of liquid green-yellow pus. The lymph nodes of the carcase were reactive.
Bacteriology of the lymph nodes: This showed *Streptococcus betahaemolyticus*.

Decision: Total condemnation.

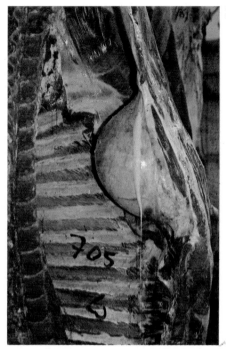

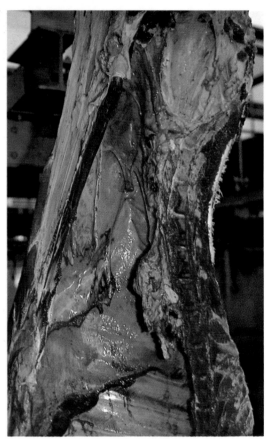

337 Fibrinous peritonitis – peritoneum: cattle An exudative inflammation of the peritoneum was observed. Extensive areas had lost their typical brightness, looking greyish. There were clots of membranous fibrin. The reaction of the lymph and renal nodes can be clearly seen.

Decision: Total condemnation.

Note: If no reactive lymph nodes are found and if there is no effect on the general condition of the meat, the decision may be approval or approval conditioned to thermal treatment, after elimination of the affected tissues. Encapsulated abscesses of the peritoneum allow for a decision of approval with elimination of the affected tissues.

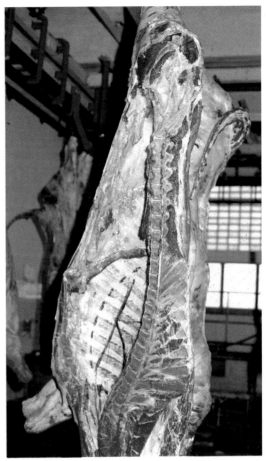

338 Purulent peritonitis – peritoneum: cattle
Acute inflammation affects the parietal peritoneum.
A purulent yellow exudate formed, which can be
seen in extensive areas of the serosa.

Decision: Total condemnation.

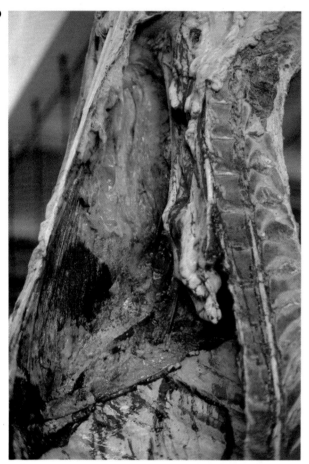

339   Fibrinopurulent peritonitis – peritoneum: cattle
The surface of the parietal sheath of the peritoneum, which
was highly congested and finely granular, was covered by a
greenish-yellow fibrinous purulent matter.

Decision: Total condemnation.

340 **Pearl disease (tuberculosis)
– peritoneum: cattle** Numerous
tuberculous lesions in the
peritoneum continue up to the
pelvis.

Differential diagnosis:
Actinobacillosis; Chronic
peritonitis; Mesothelioma.

Decision: Total condemnation.

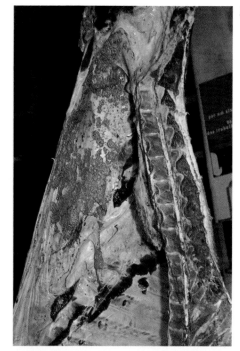

341 **Pearl disease
(tuberculosis) –
peritoneum: cattle** The
serosa covering the
rumen showed many
nodular tuberculous
lesions which occur
slowly during the course
of the disease.

Decision: Total
condemnation.

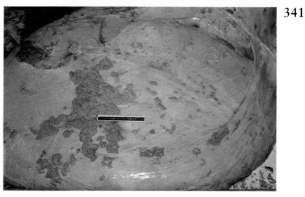

342   Chronic peritonitis –
peritoneum: cattle   The parietal
serosa showed non-specific lesions of
chronic peritonitis resembling pearl
disease. Histopathological
examination revealed a chronic
inflammatory reaction with marked
infiltration by histiocytes and
eosinophils, suggesting a parasitic
aetiology.

Differential diagnosis: Pearl disease
(tuberculosis); Mesothelioma.

Decision: Approval with elimination
of the affected tissues.

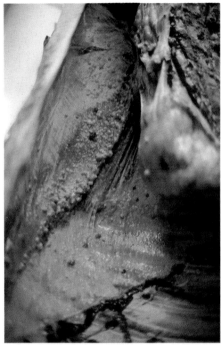

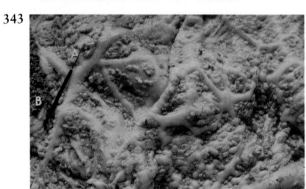

343   Chronic
peritonitis (peritoneum):
cattle   Close-up on the
chronic peritonitis
shown in **342**.
A: sectioned nodule.
B: mucosa of the rumen.

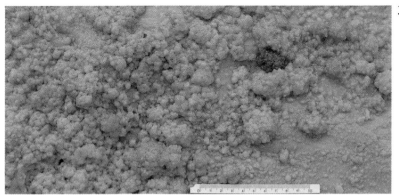

344 Chronic peritonitis, assuming a papillomatous appearance: cattle The parietal serosa was almost covered with cauliflower-like nodules, as a result of a chronic inflammatory reaction.

Differential diagnosis: Tuberculous peritonitis (pearl disease); Mesothelioma.

Decision: Approval with elimination of the affected tissues.

345 Mesothelioma – parietal peritoneum: cattle The transverse splitting of the carcase made just behind the diaphragm showed that the serosa over it was diffusely affected by a mesothelioma. This tumour which was confined to the abdominal cavity of a young heifer, did not affect the thoracic cavity.

Differential diagnosis: Pearl disease (tuberculosis); Actinobacillosis; Peritonitis by trematodes.

Decision: Total condemnation. Asbestos is considered as the aetiological agent of mesotheliomas, according to the results and conclusions of the International Agency for Research on Cancer and referred to in its *Monographs on the Evaluation of the Carcinogenic Risk of Chemicals to Humans.*

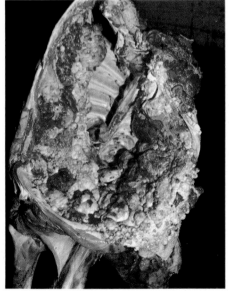

346

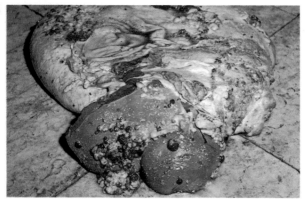

346 Mesothelioma – visceral peritoneum: cattle The surface of the serosa covering the abdominal viscera was seeded with small round nodules, yellow-white or red. When sectioned they were lardaceous and shiny which suggested their neoplastic nature.

Differential diagnosis: Pearl disease (tuberculosis); Actinobacillosis; Chronic peritonitis.

Decision: Total condemnation.

Mesentery and omentum

347

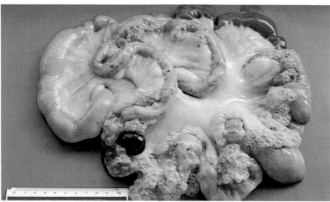

347 Emphysema of the mesentery: swine At the lower part of the intestine, particularly where it meets the mesentery, numerous transparent vesicles were seen, containing only air. It is thought that the cause for such a problem may be some strains of *E. coli*, whose great capacity for fermentating sugars, lead to the production of gas which would accumulate in the lymphatics.

Decision: Approval with elimination of the intestine.

348 Umbilical hernia – omentum: swine A large umbilical hernia was identified in the ante-mortem inspection of a swine. The content of the hernia consisted of a tissue assuming the shape of cords of round section, resulting from a chronic inflammatory reaction of the mesentery, which also affected the omentum.

Differential diagnosis: Omphalophlebitis; Cyst; Neoplasia.

Decision: Approval with elimination of the affected tissues.

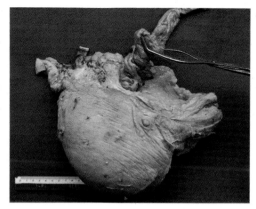

349 Haematoma – mesentery: cattle A considerable spherical swelling was located in the mesentery and showed externally a red-brown colour. The incision showed it contained dark-red almost black coagulated blood.

Differential diagnosis: Neoplasia.

Decision: Approval with elimination of the affected tissues.

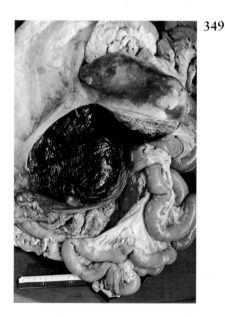

350

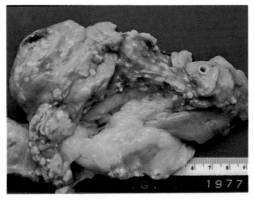

350 **Necrosis of the abdominal fat – omentum: swine** Numerous white necrotic foci of various shapes were identified in the fat of the omentum.

Decision: Approval with elimination of the affected omentum.

351

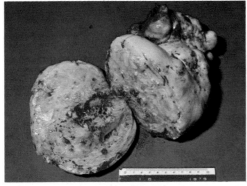

351 **Chondro-osteoma – omentum: horse** The opening of the abdominal cavity showed in the omentum, at the linea alba, a round encapsulated neoplasia, with a humped profile and firm consistency. It was easy to cut but the central tissues were particularly hard and gritty.

Decision: Approval with elimination of the neoplasia.

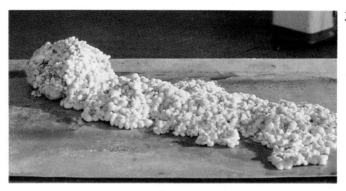

352 Lipoma – omentum: horse This massive yellow neoplasia, 2 m long, was located in the abdominal cavity of a horse. The neoplastic tissue was formed of small rounded nodules, greasy to the touch.

Decision: Approval with elimination of the neoplasia.

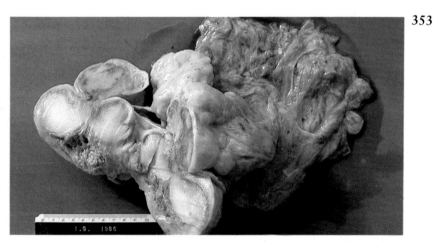

353 Fibrolipoma – mesentery: horse Multinodular neoplasia originated from a horse mesentery. The cut surface of the nodules showed firm consistency, butter-yellow colour and greasy to touch.

Differential diagnosis: Malignant tumours.

Decision: Approval with elimination of the tumour.

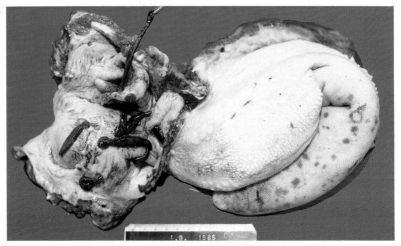

354   Parasites – mouth (oropharynx): cattle   A few leeches, haematophagous parasites are attached to the pharynx and larynx.
Parasitological examination: Limnatis nilotica.

Decision: Approval with elimination of the parasites and the tissues eventually affected.

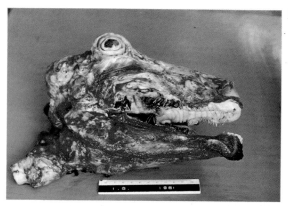

355 Fibroepithelioma – gums: sheep The swelling of the tissues of the right cheek was due to a neoplasia which grew from the gum. A molar tooth was missing and neoplastic tissue invaded the dental alveolus.

Differential diagnosis: Dental caries; parodontitis.

Decision: Total condemnation.

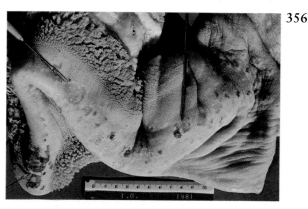

356 Aphthous rumenitis (type C virus) – rumen: cattle The eroded areas in the mucosa resulted from ruptured vesicles that are very frequently formed in ruminants affected by foot and mouth disease.

Decision: Total condemnation.

5: The circulatory system

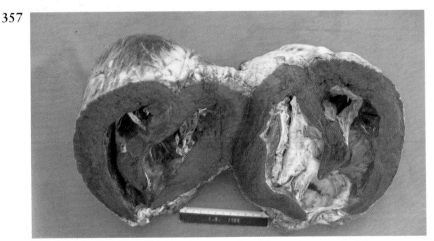

357 Congenital disturbance – heart: cattle The exploratory incision – determined by the abnormal heartshape – revealed two congenital malformations. One was an interruption of the cardiac muscle in the ventricular wall, the cavity being kept closed by the visceral pericardium and by the endocardium. The second malformation was a wide interventricular communication, due to incomplete development of the interventricular septum.

Decision: Approval with elimination of the heart.

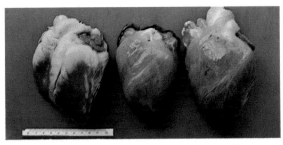

358 Hydrocachexia – epicardial fat: sheep The heart shown in the centre and on the right are examples of hydrocachexia; a normal heart is on the left. The heart in the centre showed the normal fat replaced by a gelatinous fluidified fat, while in the heart on the right small areas of normal fat could still be seen.

Decision: The meat of the carcases corresponding to the hearts in the centre and on the right was totally condemned due to hydrocachexia.

359 Haemopericardium: cattle

Considerable haemopericardium is visible, as well as colour modification. The condition was due to the accumulation of fibrin and coagulated blood over the visceral pericardium.

Decision: Approval, if no other lesions are found, with elimination of the heart.

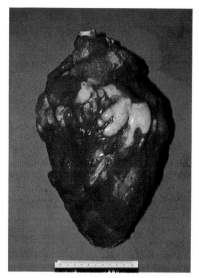

359

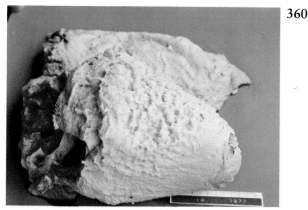

360

360 Fibrinous pericarditis – pericardium: cattle The surface of the heart is fully covered by a fibrinous matter of soft consistency and yellow colour, which also extends into the parietal pericardium.

Decision: Approval, if no other lesions are found, with elimination of the heart.

Diseases of the pericardium, heart and vessels: criteria for post-mortem inspection

Pericarditis
(a) Total condemnation:
    (i) in cases of acute infectious exudative pericarditis;
    (ii) if signs of septicaemia are present and in cases of bovine traumatic pericarditis with fever;
    (iii) in cases of large accumulation of exudate, circulatory disturbances, degenerative changes in organs or abnormal odour.
(b) Approval conditioned to thermal treatment (kH), subject to laboratory examination and with elimination of the heart and affected parts of the carcase, in cases of subacute infectious exudative pericarditis.
(c) Approved with elimination of the heart and affected parts of the carcase:
    (i) in cases of chronic infectious pericarditis, without complications, in well-nourished animals;
    (ii) in cases of chronic bovine traumatic pericarditis.

Endocarditis
(a) Total condemnation:
    In cases of verrucose endocarditis with circulatory disturbances in the lungs or liver, with recent infiltration and in animals showing general debility.
(b) Approval conditioned to thermal treatment (kH), with elimination of the heart:
    In cases of ulcerative and verrucose endocarditis, without complications.
(c) Approval with elimination of the heart:
    In cases of fully cicatrized endocarditis.

Heart lesions of a non-infectious nature
Approval with elimination of the heart.

361

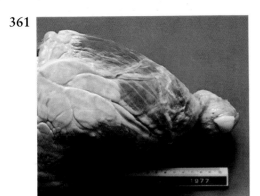

361 Abscess attached to the heart apex – pericardium: cattle A round nodule is attached to the visceral pericardium. Incision revealed an abscess of thick fibrous wall, with creamy yellowish-grey pus. Lesions of fibrinous pericarditis could be seen in the area around the apex.

Differential diagnosis: Neoplasia.

Decision: Approval with elimination of the heart.

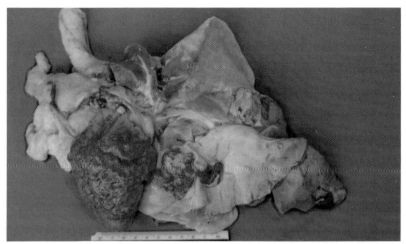

362 Fibrinohaemorrhagic pericarditis – pericardium: sheep The visceral pericardium is affected by an acute exudative inflammation. The internal face of the parietal pericardium showed small inflammatory foci with similar characteristics. The lungs were equally affected.

Decision: Total condemnation or approval conditioned to thermal treatment, subject to the results of the laboratory examination.

363 Purulent pericarditis – pericardium: cattle The profile of the heart was irregular due to a purulent pericarditis. The parietal serosa was equally affected by a chronic inflammatory process with fibrous evolution. The corresponding carcase presented signs of septicaemia.

Differential diagnosis: Tuberculosis.

Decision: Total condemnation.

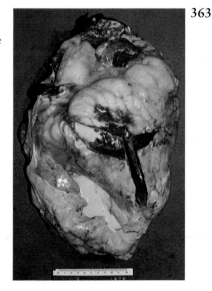

363

364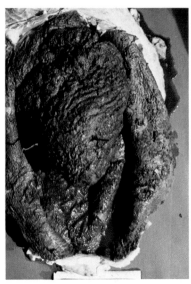

364 Traumatic pericarditis: cattle The thickened pericardium was affected by a chronic inflammatory reaction whose traumatic nature is clearly visible in the picture. The perforating body migrated up to the myocardium, causing a large haemorrhage. The blood accumulated in the pericardium. Signs of traumatic pericarditis were found in the carcase and the thorax had a fetid odour.

Decision: Total condemnation.

365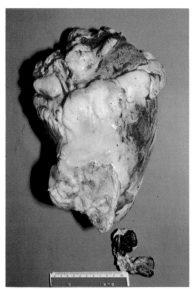

365 Chronic pericarditis – pericardium: cattle An exudative inflammatory reaction has led to the deposition of fibrin in the pericardial cavity. During the subsequent organization of the exudate, adherences were formed between the two layers which explain the irregular profile of the heart.

Differential diagnosis: Tuberculosis.

Decision: Approval with elimination of the heart.

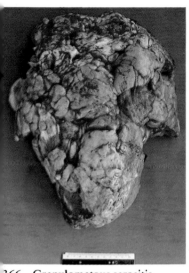

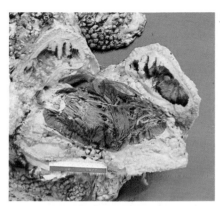

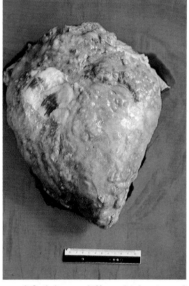

366 Granulomatous serositis (tuberculosis) – pericardium: cattle Large areas of newly formed inflammatory tissue can be seen over the pericardium. Caseation is not usually present, but whenever it occurs, shows up as fine streaks. These are the changes characteristic of the chronic tuberculosis of the heart. The lymph nodes were affected.

Differential diagnosis: Chronic non-specific pericarditis; Neoplasia.

Decision: Total condemnation.

367 Diffuse caseating serositis (tuberculosis) – pericardium: cattle The lesions of diffuse caseating serositis are typical of the breakdown of body resistance, the visceral serosa being affected by a specific exudative inflammation.

Decision: Total condemnation.

368 Granulomatous serositis (tuberculosis) – pericardium: cattle The profile of the heart was modified due to diffuse thickening of the pericardium. The heart was yellowish-white with small, prominent, hard, yellow nodules of caseous necrosis, complicated with calcification.

Differential diagnosis: Non-specific pericarditis.

Decision: Total condemnation.

203

369

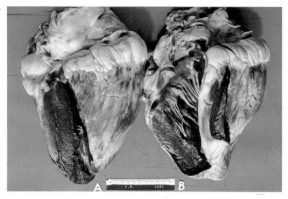

369 Brown atrophy – heart: cattle The heart labelled A looks normal in contrast with the heart labelled B which shows a dark-brown colour, due to the intracytoplasmic deposition of lipofuscins, usually named age pigment.

Differential diagnosis: Melanosis.

Decision: Approval with elimination of the atrophic heart.

370

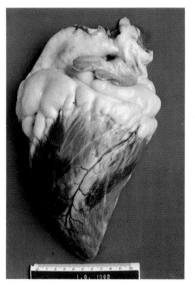

370 Melanosis – heart: cattle Several black stains of different sizes were present in the heart muscle, under the pericardium, due to disturbed melanogenesis. Identical changes could be seen in the lungs, pleura, kidneys, blood vessels and lymph nodes.

Decision: Total condemnation due to generalisation.

371 Lipomatosis – heart: cattle The heart, affected by a degenerative disease, presented a whitish-yellow colour. The degenerative changes were also seen inside the cardiac muscle.

Differential diagnosis: Zenker's degeneration.

Decision: Approval with elimination of the heart.

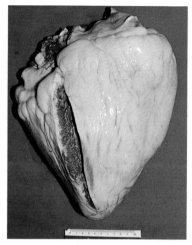
371

372 Xanthomatosis – heart: horse The fat around the coronary vessels was orange and the same abnormal colour was noticed in the carcase.

Differential diagnosis: Brown atrophy.

Decision: Total condemnation due to generalisation.

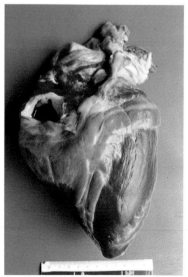
372

205

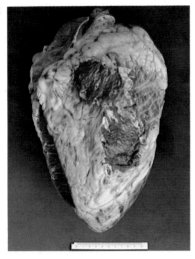

373 Hypertrophy and dilated blood vessels – heart: cattle The heart was yellowish and at the surface a series of sma ampullar swellings could be noticed under the pericardium. The incision of the myocardium revealed a series of small cavities corresponding to dilatations of small subepicardial vessels whose wall presented an hypertrophic muscular layer.

Decision: Approval with elimination of the heart.

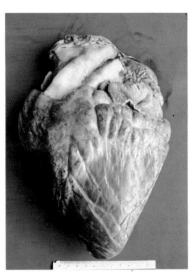

374 Petechial haemorrhages – heart: cattle In the fat of the coronary groove and longitudinal groove numerous petechiae could be noticed.

Differential diagnosis: Poisoning by pesticides; Pasteurellosis; Anthrax; Asphyxia.

Decision: Approval with elimination of the heart if no other lesions are found.

375 Petechial haemorrhages – heart: cattle Numerous subepicardial haemorrhages in the ventricle. These are frequently found in cases of multiple slaughtering haemorrhages.

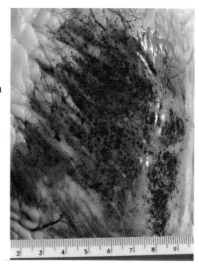

Differential diagnosis: Haemorrhages from poisoning; Septicaemia; Rinderpest; Anaphylaxis.

Decision: Approval with elimination of the heart if no other lesions are found.

376 Myocardial infarct or focal necrotic myocarditis – heart: cattle The post-mortem inspection of the heart revealed a greyish area of well-defined limits, surrounded by a whitish-yellow halo. The incision showed a grey tissue of spongy consistency, due to ischaemia following a coronary obliteration.

Differential diagnosis: Metastasis of neoplasia.

Decision: Approval with elimination of the heart.

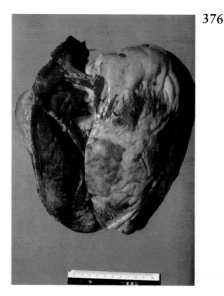

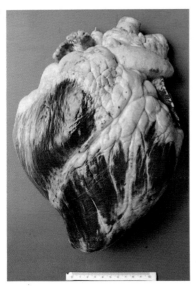

377 **377 Myocardial degeneration – heart: cattle** Degeneration of the myocardium, probably of circulatory origin, revealed by a brownish colour with purple reflexes of the muscle. A few sarcosporidian cysts can be seen under the visceral serosa.

Differential diagnosis: Brown atrophy; Melanosis.

Decision: Approval, if no other lesions are found, with elimination of the heart.

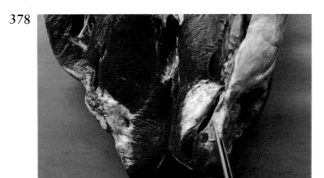

378

378 Myocardial degeneration – heart: cattle A degeneration of the myocardium located near the apex leading to the total disappearance of the muscular fibres. The ventricular wall was reduced to a delicate fibrous lamina, covered by the epicardium and endocardium.

Differential diagnosis: Metastasis of neoplasia.

Decision: Approval with elimination of the heart's affected tissue.

379 Focal necrotic myocarditis – heart: cattle Necropurulent foci of regular limits in the myocardium, which also showed colour changes in some restricted areas due to degeneration of the fibres.

Differential diagnosis: Metastasis of neoplasia.

Decision: Total condemnation or, alternatively, approval conditioned to thermal treatment, according to results of laboratory examination, with elimination of the heart.

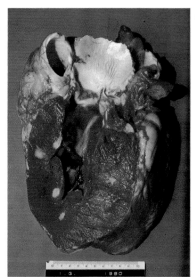

379

380 Subacute myocarditis – heart: cattle In the upper wall of the right ventricle, there was a pale area, with rounded limits, slightly prominent. Incisions in that area showed changes in the structure of the myocardium due to a hard white tissue with some small haemorrhages.

Differential diagnosis: Metastasis of neoplasia.

Decision: Approval subject to thermal treatment, and the results of laboratory examinations, with elimination of the heart.

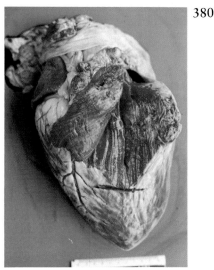

380

381

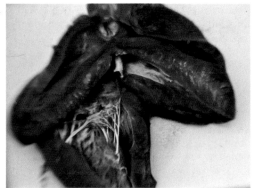

381 Necrotic myocarditis (foot and mouth disease) – heart: cattle Foci of discoloration were particularly abundant in the ventricles. Incision revealed numerous pale stripes with the typical appearance of the so-called tiger-heart.

Decision: Total condemnation

382

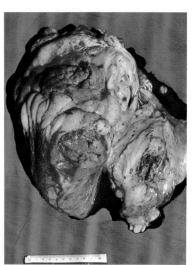

382 Traumatic myocarditis – heart: cattle In the left ventricle wall, slightly above the apex of the heart, the myocardium presented a greenish colour in an area where the pericardium sheaths were adherent. The incision showed a purulent passage, surrounded by a fibrous inflammatory reaction, due to the action of a perforating foreign body.

Decision: Total condemnation or, alternatively, approval conditioned to thermal treatment, with elimination of the heart, subject to the results of the laboratory examinations.

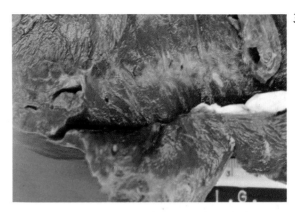

383 Chronic myocarditis – heart: cattle The heart showed subepicardial areas of discoloration, which the incision showed to be due to the replacement of the muscle fibres for a whitish-yellow fibrous tissue.

Differential diagnosis: Necrotic myocarditis of foot and mouth disease.

Decision: Approval with elimination of the heart.

384 Myocardial cicatrisation – heart: cattle The longitudinal section of the left ventricle revealed two areas of irregular profile, whitish-yellow, shiny and 2 cm in diameter. The consistency was firm and they were hard to cut.

Differential diagnosis: Metastasis of neoplasia.

Decision: Approval with elimination of the affected tissues.

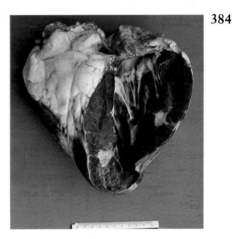

385

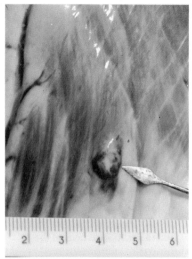

385 Sarcosporidiasis – heart: cattle
Inserted in the ventricular muscle, a small white elliptical body could be seen, prominent under the epicardium. It was a *Sarcocystis* cyst.

Differential diagnosis: Cysticercosis; Toxoplasmosis.

Decision: Approval, if no other lesions are found, with elimination of the heart.

386

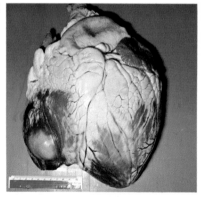

386 Hydatid cyst – heart: cattle In the wall of the right ventricle there was a large cyst with a thin transparent wall, characteristic of the hydatid cyst. The location is rather infrequent.

Decision: Approval with elimination of the heart.

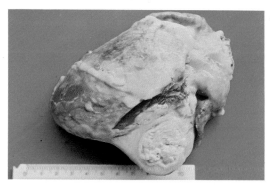

387 Hydatid cyst – heart: sheep The incision of a reduced swelling in a ventricle wall revealed a purulent, greenish hydatid cyst. It was completely isolated from the myocardium by fibrous tissue.

Decision: Approval with elimination of the heart.

388 Parasitic myocarditis (cysticercosis) – heart: cattle The incision of the myocardium showed some thick, fibrous cysts whose inner walls were calcified. The cysts contained solidified yellowish necrotic matter.

Differential diagnosis: Sarcosporidiosis; Toxoplasmosis.

Decision: Approval, conditional to thermal treatment at 60°C. (140°F.), in the centre of the meat, with elimination of the heart.

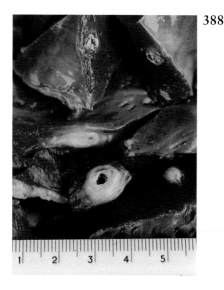

389

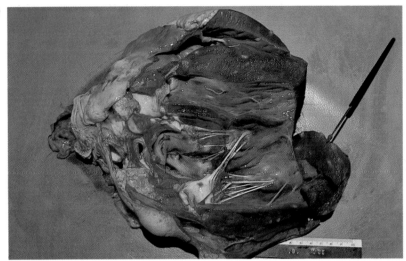

389   Parasitic myocarditis (cysticercosis) – heart: cattle   Under the parietal serosa of the pericardium, clear elliptical formations were observed, slightly protruding. The incision of the organ showed a few identical structures in the myocardium. These were vesicles of *Cysticercus bovis*, the larval stage of the *Taenia saginata*.

Differential diagnosis: Sarcosporidiosis; Metastasis from neoplasia; Focal myocarditis.

Decision: Approval, conditional to thermal treatment at 60°C., in the centre of the meat, with elimination of the heart (moderate infection).

390

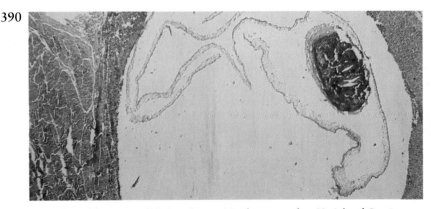

390   Parasitic myocarditis (cysticercosis) – heart: cattle   Vesicle of *Cysticercus bovis* with a scolex in development stage. H. & E.

391 Rhabdomyoma – heart: cattle A considerable neoplasia multilobulated and pearly, attached to the ventricular wall.

Differential diagnosis:
Rhabdomyosarcoma; Neurofibroma.

Decision: Approval with elimination of the heart.

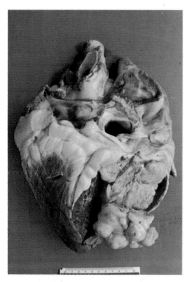

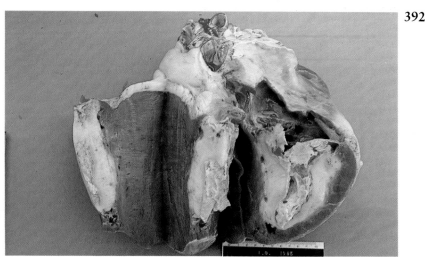

392 Fibrosarcoma – heart: cattle Underlying necrotic purulent lesions of the endocardium a connective tissue neoplasia was formed, showing milky-white coloration and firm consistency.

Decision: Total condemnation.

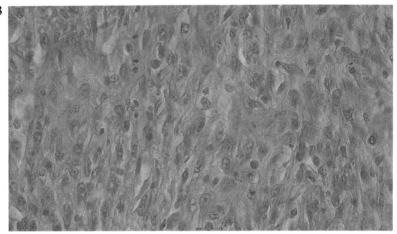

393 Fibrosarcoma – heart: cattle Underneath a lesion of vegetative endocarditis, a fibrosarcoma developed in the myocardium, probably arising from the highly cellular connective tissue which was the origin of the inflammatory lesions of the endocardium. H. & E.

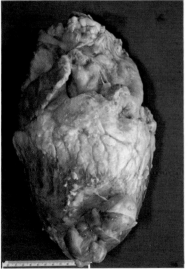

394 Rhabdomyosarcoma – heart: cattle A neoplasia was attached to the external wall of the left ventricle, near the apex of the heart. The tumour, which deformed the ventricle, was attached to a broad pedicle and was made of a tissue identical to muscle, light-brown and shiny. Its structure was homogeneous.

Differential diagnosis: Rhabdomyoma; Tuberculosis; Neurofibroma.

Decision: Total condemnation.

395 Metastasis of a splenic sarcoma – heart: horse Several nodules at the surface of the heart under the epicardium. They comprised lardaceous yellowish tissue, disseminated within the myocardium. A few nodules were also identified in the auricles.

Differential diagnosis: Neurofibromatosis; focal necrotic myocarditis.

Decision: Total condemnation.

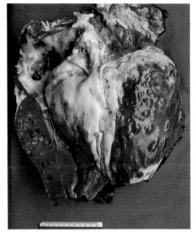

396 Melanoblastoma – heart: horse At the ventricular septum, near the apex of the heart, two black nodules were located, shiny and irregular, corresponding to the metastatic dissemination of a melanoblastoma.

Decision: Total condemnation.

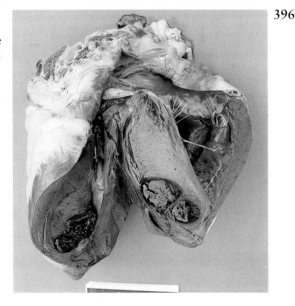

397

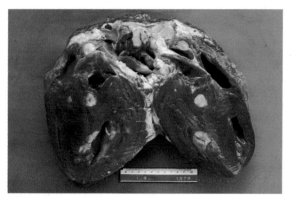

397 Metastasis of a kidney adenocarcinoma – heart: horse   Within the myocardium, in the ventricular wall, several well-defined whitish nodules of various sizes were identified. They had a homogeneous structure resembling immature connective tissue.

Differential diagnosis: Focal necrotic myocarditis.

Decision: Total condemnation.

398

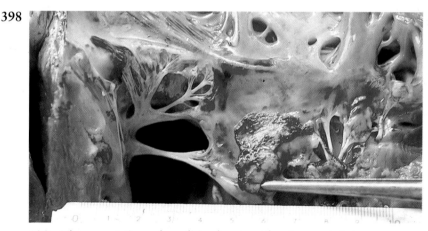

398 Ulcerovegetative endocarditis – heart: cattle   A necrotic lesion was located in the tricuspid valve, which was thickened and highly congested in that area.

Decision: Approval conditioned to thermal treatment, subject to the results of the laboratory examination, with elimination of the heart.

399 Verrucous endocarditis – heart: cattle In the tricuspid valve a large necrotic mass was formed, very friable, yellow and looking like a cauliflower, with congestive haemorrhagic areas. These valvular diseases frequently disturb the venous circulation and are responsible for the dissemination of the agent to the lungs.

Decision: Total condemnation or approval, subject to thermal treatment, with elimination of the heart, subject to laboratory examination.

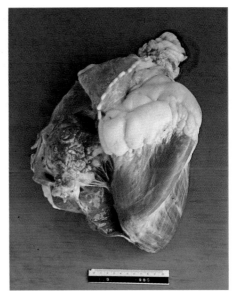

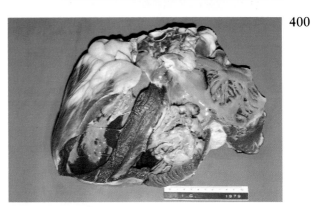

400 Verrucous endocarditis – heart: cattle The bicuspid valve was affected by an inflammatory reaction which produced large amounts of yellow-greenish necrotic material, extremely friable. This occupied most of the ventricle. Simultaneously, several organs showed congestive changes.

Decision: Total condemnation.

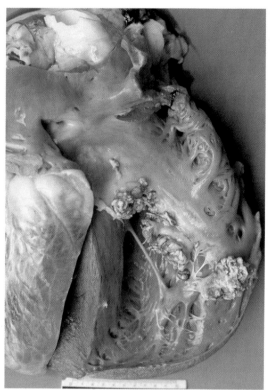

**401 Verrucous valvular endocarditis (with
complications) – heart: cattle** An endocarditis of
undetermined aetiology developed in the tricuspid valve,
which posteriorly evolved towards a self-maintained
condition leading to the formation and deposition of
immune complexes.

Decision: Total condemnation.

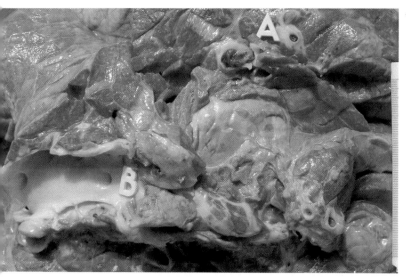

402 Complications of verrucous endocarditis (septic embolism) – lung: cattle (Same case as **401**.) In some of the branches of the pulmonary artery, an endarteritis process developed, as a consequence of the embolism of material which detached from the tricuspid valve endocarditis.

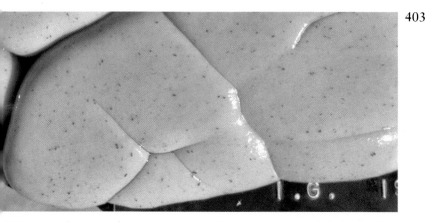

403 Complications of verrucous endocarditis (suppurative embolic nephritis) – kidney: cattle (Same case as **401**.) Small congestive haemorrhagic foci can be seen at the surface of the kidney, due to the embolism of pyogenic microorganisms in the glomerular corpuscle.

404

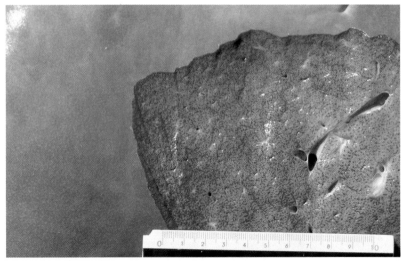

404　Complications of verrucous endocarditis (chronic passive congestion) – liver: cattle　(Same case as **401**.) Stasis of blood was noticed in the central veins, causing a deep red colour which contrasted with the periphery of the lobules. These changes are a consequence of the organic and functional disturbances of the tricuspid valve.

405

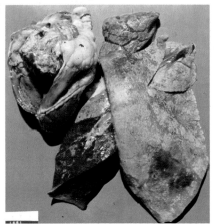

405　Mural endocarditis – heart: sheep　The wall of the right auricle showed a considerable yellow necrotic mass that filled most of the cavity. Metastatic foci could be seen in the lungs, due to embolism of the bacteria coming from the heart lesions.

Decision: Total condemnation.

406 Hydatid cyst – heart: cattle The incision of the left ventricle revealed a large hydatid cyst originating in the endocardium, that filled most of the ventricular cavity.

The heart is pale because it was submitted to fixation in 10% formalin.

Decision: Approval with elimination of the heart.

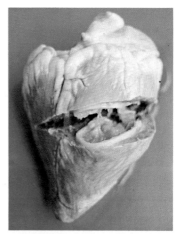

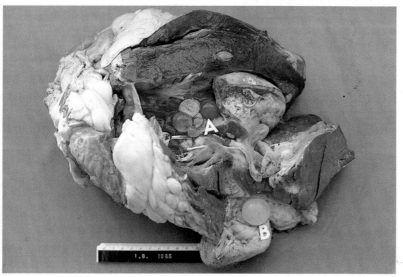

407 Hydatid cyst – heart: cattle The exploratory incision of the heart showed a hydatid cyst inserted in the endocardium of the right ventricle, which compressed the wall of the left ventricle. The accidental opening of the cyst showed numerous daughter cysts.

Decision: Approval with elimination of the heart.

408

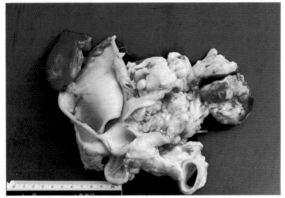

408 Thrombus – fragment of aorta: cattle The accidental opening of the aorta revealed, in the lumbar region, a round mass, red and dull approximately 5 cm in diameter. As it was friable and adherent to the intima of the vessel, in an area where the endothelium was damaged, it was thought to be a thrombus.

Differential diagnosis: Carcinoma of the adrenal medulla.

Decision: Approval.

409

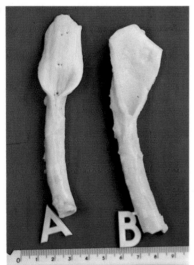

409 Jaundice – fragment of aorta: sheep Two fragments of abdominal aorta are shown in the picture. The organ in B was infiltrated with biliary pigments, in contra to the normal fragment shown in A.

Differential diagnosis: Pigmentation by trypaflavine, atabrine or picric acid.

Decision: Total condemnation of the case shown in B.

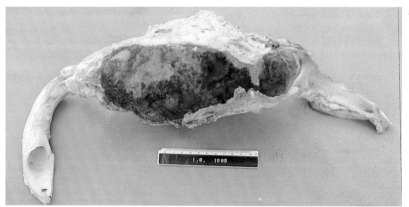

410   Aneurysm – sections of aorta: cattle   The abdominal aorta, near the kidney, presented a marked increase in its diameter. The large spindle-shaped aneurysm, 30 cm in diameter, was calcified and it fractured at the splitting of the carcase.

Decision: Approval with elimination of the affected blood vessel.

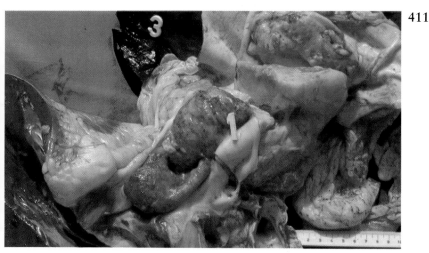

411   Obliterating thrombophlebitis – posterior vena cava: cattle   Along a large extension of the posterior vena cava, the changes due to a thrombophlebitis were quite evident, with almost complete obstruction of the vessel by a solid mass, encephaloid-like, more or less congested, which was at the origin of the cardiac liver lesions, also noticeable in the picture.

Decision: Total condemnation, due to severe circulatory disturbance.

412

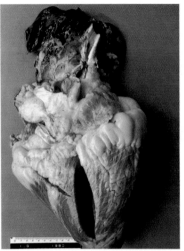

412 Melanotic sarcoma – aorta: cattle
Closely surrounding the adventitia of the aorta, near the origin of the vessel, a firm, black and shiny neoplasia was identified.

Differential diagnosis: Blood clot.

Decision: Total condemnation.

413

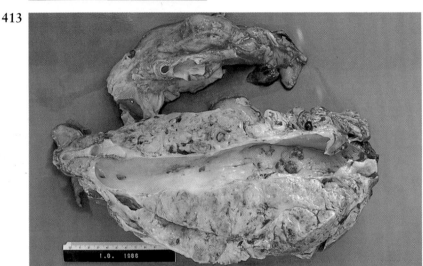

413 Metastasis from an epidermoid carcinoma of the lung – fragment of aorta: cattle The wall of the abdominal aorta was externally invaded by a neoplasia originating in the lung. The tumour which also affected other smaller arteries destroyed the aortic wall in some areas and it was clearly apparent in the lumen as sessile round vegetations.

Decision: Total condemnation.

6: The haematopoietic organs:

Lymph nodes

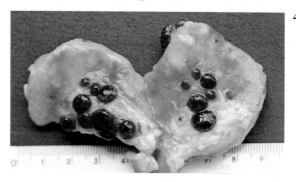

414   Haemal nodes included in the superficial cervical lymph node: sheep   Although infrequent, these findings should be considered normal.

Differential diagnosis: Focal haemorrhages in the lymph node; Metastasis of neoplasias.

Decision: Approval with elimination of the organ (for aesthetic reasons).

415   Anthracosis (and metastasis of carcinoma) – lymph node: cattle   The bronchial lymph node was easily recognized due to the presence of coal dust (anthracosis), particularly along the convex surface of the organ. This was completely invaded by metastasis of a tumour (carcinoma) which gave it a typical homogeneous and shiny appearance.

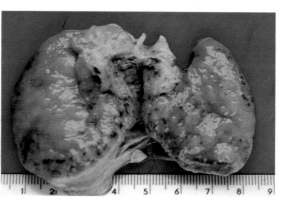

Decision: Total condemnation. Anthracosis alone involves elimination of the affected organs.

416

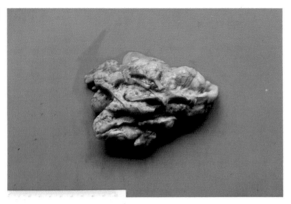

416 Polycystic lymph node: cattle The organ was bosselated by numerous cysts, containing a lymph-like fluid, caused by a deficient circulation of lymph in the lymph node.

Decision: Approval with elimination of the organ.

417

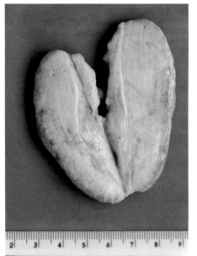

417 Emphysema – superficial cervical lymph node: cattle The lymph node was considerably enlarged, and when sectioned revealed a discrete crepitation. The cut surface was dry and yellow. Cause: the accumulation of gas within the organ, as a consequence of subcutaneous insufflation of air to facilitate the removal of the skin.

Decision: Approval, if bacteriological examination is negative.
Subcutaneous insufflation is nowadays forbidden in many countries. In cases of marked emphysema the lymph nodes float in water.

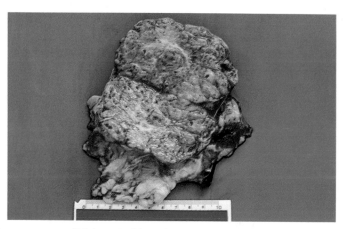

418 Emphysema – superficial cervical lymph node: cattle The organ was bosselated with a spongy consistency. It revealed, when sectioned, a crepitation caused by accumulation of gas inside small cavities.

Differential diagnosis: Emphysema due to subcutaneous insufflation of air.

Decision: Approval, if no other lesions are found, with elimination of the organ. Laboratory tests are necessary if the lesion is generalized, affecting other lymph nodes.

419

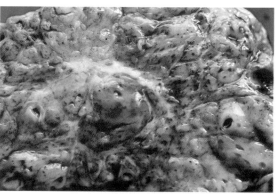

419 Emphysema – superficial cervical lymph node: cattle Magnification of an area of lymph node from case shown in **418**. The small cavities can be easily seen.

420

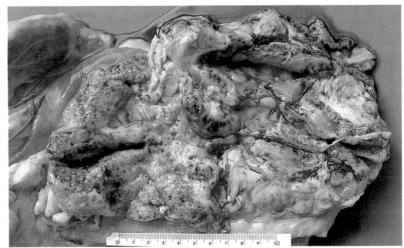

420 Emphysema – mediastinal lymph nodes: cattle The mediastinal lymph nodes show anthracosis and are hypertrophic due to numerous vesicles of non-odorous and colourless gas. The same process had taken place in other lymph nodes.

Bacteriological examination: This showed *Clostridium perfrigens*.

Differential diagnosis: Emphysema due to subcutaneous inflation of air.

Decision: Total condemnation.

421

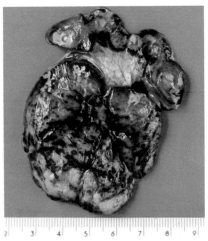

421 Acute lymphadenitis – iliac lymp node: swine The incision of the organ showed a hyperplastic lymphoid tissue and many small haemorrhagic foci.

Decision: Approval, if no other lesions found, with elimination of the organ. The decision is subject to the spread of process and to the existence and nature lesions in the tissues drained by the lym node.

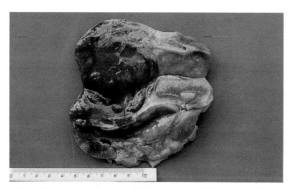

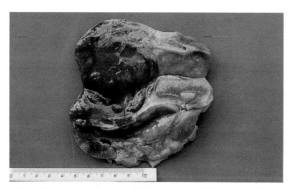
422

422   Hyperreactive condition – superficial cervical lymph node: cattle   The enlarged lymph node was affected by a reactive process revealed by congestive haemorrhagic lesions, together with marked hyperplasia of the lymphoid tissue.

Decision: Approval, if no other lesions are found, with elimination of the organ.

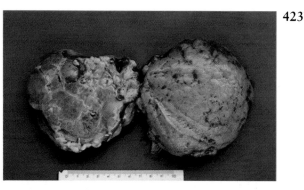
423

423   Non-specific acute lymphadenitis – iliac lymph node: cattle   The lymph node was very much enlarged due to the hyperplasia of the lymphoid tissue, which presented a thin granular yellow-pink cut surface, with small congestive haemorrhagic foci.

Decision: Approval with elimination of the organ.
Note: The area drained did not show any lesions.

424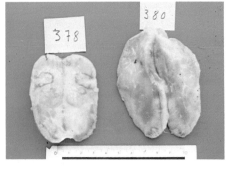

424 Non-specific acute lymphadenitis – superficial cervical lymph nodes: cattle

Differential diagnosis: Lymphoid hyperplasia and infarct type lesions; Hypertrophic, oedematous and congestive lymph nodes.

These organs were removed from a carcase of an animal with general systemic reaction, resulting from methylthiouracil administration.

Decision: Total condemnation.
Note: Apart from lymphadenitis, changes were also noted in the thyroid, adrenal gland, and testes. There was an increase of the content of free water in the meat.

425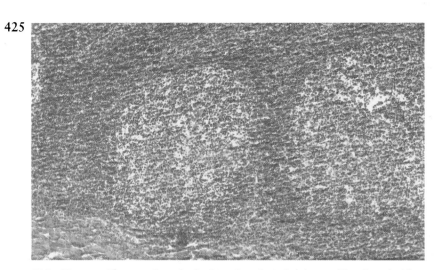

425 Non-specific acute lymphadenitis – lymph node: sheep Two lymphoid nodules can be seen in the cortex, with large pale centres, surrounded by reticular tissue, with the sinuses partially obstructed with erythrocytes. These changes are identifiable with a non-specific acute lymphadenitis. H. & E.

426   Non-specific acute lymphadenitis – superficial cervical lymph node: cattle   Acute lymphadenitis due to traumatic lesions during transport. The organ was moist with dispersed haemorrhages.

Differential diagnosis: lymphadenitis (a) due to chemicals; (b) due to infectious diseases.

Decision: Approval, if no other lesions are found.

Note: The area drained by this lymph node presented traumatic lesions which were therefore eliminated together with the lymph node.

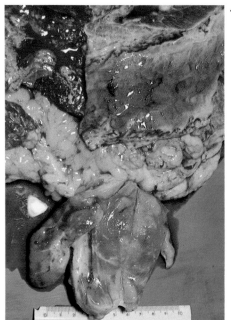

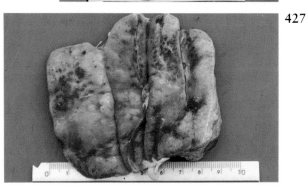

427   Non-specific acute lymphadenitis – lymph node: cattle   A clear hyperplasia of the cortex of the lymph node associated with congestive haemorrhagic lesions, both indicating acute inflammation.

428

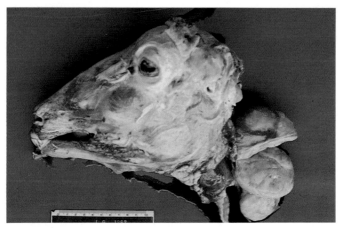

428 Non-specific acute lymphadenitis – retropharyngeal lymph node: sheep The lymph node was markedly hypertrophic and the cut surface was shiny and moist.

Differential diagnosis: Lymphoid leukosis.

Decision: Approval, if no other lesions are found, with elimination of the head and tongue.

429

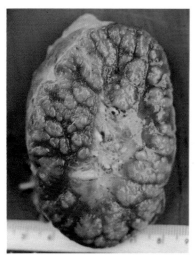

429 Non-specific acute lymphadenitis – lumbar lymph node: cattle The lymph node was enlarged, congested, with a shiny cut surface. The hyperplastic lymphoid tissue was slightly prominent. There was generalized lymphadenitis.

Bacteriological examination: Showed *Staphylococcus coagulase* + and *Streptococcus betahaemolyticus.*

Decision: Total condemnation due to generalized lymphadenitis.

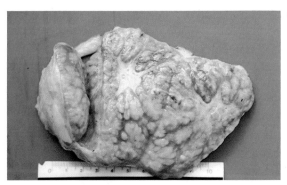

430   Non-specific acute lymphadenitis – superficial inguinal lymph node: cattle   Moderate congestion and marked hyperplasia of the lymphoid tissue.

Differential diagnosis: Tuberculosis; Metastasis of neoplasias.

Decision: Approval if no other lesions are found.

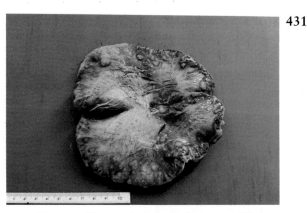

431   Non-specific acute lymphadenitis – superficial inguinal lymph node: cattle   The changes were particularly evident in the cortex. The medulla was affected by advanced sclerosis.

Decision: Approval if no other lesions are found.

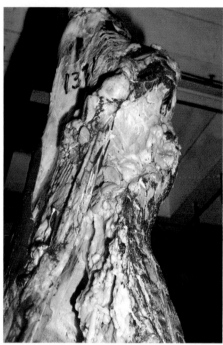

432 Non-specific acute lymphadenitis – superficial inguinal and internal iliac lymph nodes: cattle The lymph nodes were markedly hypertrophic in a case of purulent mastitis.

Decision: Total condemnation.

433 Acute lymphadenitis (African swine fever) – gastric lymph nodes: swine The gastric lymph nodes were hypertrophic with oedema and focal haemorrhages, particularly clear in the cortex of the organ. African swine fever was diagnosed, although there were no symptoms ante-mortem.

Differential diagnosis: Hog cholera.

433

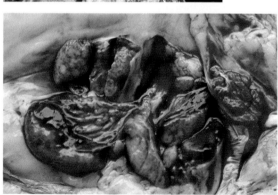

Decision: Total condemnation.
If African swine fever or hog cholera are suspected, virological and histopathological examinations are necessary. Meanwhile, carcase and offals will be held, pending laboratory examination. Animals which have been in contact with the affected swine must also be examined.

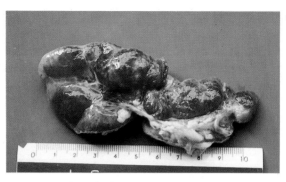

434 Acute lymphadenitis – retropharyngeal lymph node: cattle Congestion and haemorrhage were very marked in these lymph nodes – an animal which had been submitted to the action of irritant chemicals.

Bacteriological examination: This shows *Streptococcus betahaemolyticus* and *Streptococcus alphahaemolyticus*.

Decision: Approval after thermal treatment, with elimination of organs and tissues drained by these lymph nodes. In such cases, a careful inspection of the lymph nodes, lungs, liver and kidneys should be carried out.

435 Necrotic lymphadenitis – mandibular lymph node: swine The widely affected lymph node was enlarged with a moist homogeneous and shiny parenchyma, no distinction being made between cortex and medulla. A few irregular pale areas could be seen, corresponding to necrotic foci.

Decision: Approval, if no other lesions are found, with elimination of the head and tongue.

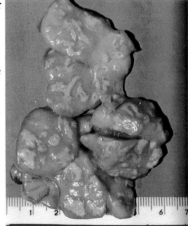

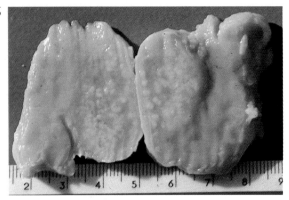

436   Necrotic lymphadenitis (contagious bovine pleuropneumonia) – bronchial lymph node: cattle
From the cut surface of this markedly hypertrophic lymph node there was a clear yellow fluid exudate, uncovering numerous small, round, pale foci, slightly prominent, which were areas of necrosis due to the action of the mycoplasm and its endotoxins.

Decision: Approval with elimination of the thoracic viscera and costal pleura.

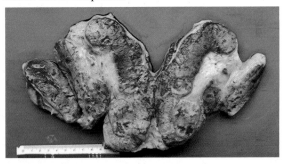

437   Necrotic lymphadenitis – superficial inguinal lymph node: cattle   The cut surface of this considerably enlarged lymph node was pink, with some dark red haemorrhages and a few greenish areas of necrosis.

Bacteriological examination: This showed *Klebsiella pneumoniae.*

Decision: Total condemnation.
Note: The iliac lymph nodes were also affected.

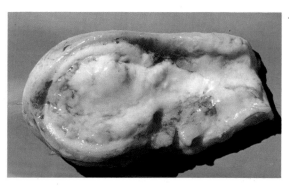

438 **Purulent lymphadenitis – bronchial lymph node: cattle** The central area of the lymph node was replaced by a homogeneous yellow purulent matter, surrounded by connective tissue isolating it from the parenchyma, which in some parts was only a few millimetres thick. Isolation of acid-alcohol fast bacilli was negative.

Decision: Approval, with elimination of the lymph node.

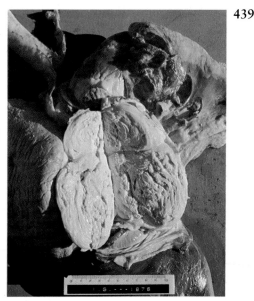

39 **Necropurulent lymphadenitis mediastinal lymph node: sheep** he enlarged lymph node was duced to the fibrous capsule and a ecrotic purulent matter which had placed the entire parenchyma.

ifferential diagnosis: Caseous berculosis.

acteriology of the pus: This showed *reptococcus betahaemolyticus.*

ecision: Approval conditional to ermal treatment, with elimination the lungs and heart.

ote: When several lymph nodes are volved or if the purulent matter esents a liquid fraction, then total ndemnation is a more suitable cision, considering the ssibility of dissemination of emolysins or bacterial organisms.

440

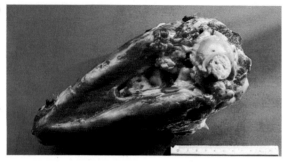

440 Purulent lymphadenitis – retropharyngeal lymph node: sheep The lymph node was enlarged due to the accumulation of a greasy greenish pus, which suggested infection by *Corynebacterium pyogenes*, confirmed by laboratory examination.

Differential diagnosis: Tuberculosis.

Decision: Approval, if no other lesions are present with elimination of the head and tongue.

441

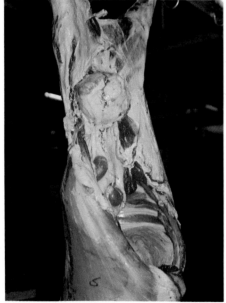

441 Infralumbar tumefaction – carcase: sheep A large tumefaction the size of a melon, of soft consistency, surrounded by a fibrous capsule.

Hypothetical diagnosis: Purulent lymphadenitis; Neoplasia; Cyst.

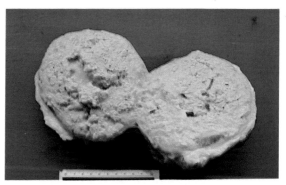

442   Purulent lymphadenitis – lumbar lymph node: sheep   Incision of the tumefaction (**441**) revealed a lymph node in which the normal tissue was replaced by a purulent greenish matter, fluidified in the central region.

Bacteriology of the pus: This showed *Streptococcus betahaemolyticus.*

Decision: Total condemnation. (See note **439**.)

443   Infralumbar tumefaction – carcase: swine
A tumefaction, the size of a melon, well encapsulated and of soft consistency.

Hypothetical diagnosis: Purulent lymphadenitis; Neoplasia; Cyst.

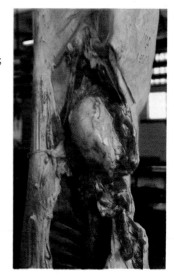

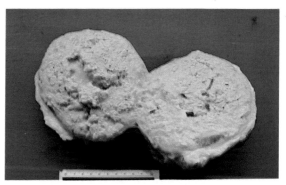

442

443

444

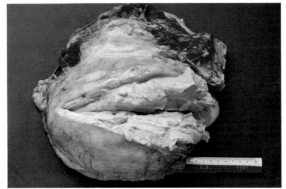

**444   Purulent lymphadenitis – lumbar lymph node:
swine**   Section of **443**. The entire parenchyma has been
replaced by a purulent greyish-yellow matter, of soft
consistency but with no signs of fluidity. This pus was
surrounded by a fibrous capsule.

Bacteriology of the pus: This showed *Streptococcus
betahaemolyticus.*

Decision: Approval after thermal treatment with
elimination of the tumefaction. (See note **439**.)

445

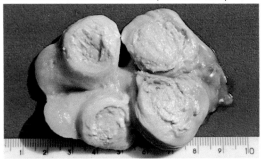

**445   Purulent lymphadenitis – popliteal lymph
node: sheep**   Abscess with a fibrous wall 3–4 mm
thick, containing greenish pasty pus.

Bacteriology of the pus: This showed
Corynebacterium ovis.

Decision: Approval, if no other lesions are present,
with elimination of the area drained by the affected
lymph node.

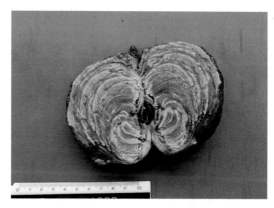

446 Caseous lymphadenitis – lymph node: sheep
Old lesion, with the typical appearance of a sectioned onion due to the action of *Corynebacterium ovis*.

Decision: Approval, if no other lesions are present, with elimination of the area drained by the affected lymph node.

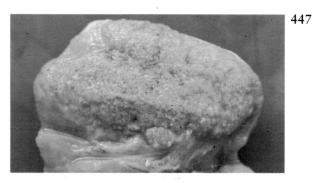

447 Tuberculosis – bronchial lymph node: cattle
Lesions of reticulated caseation, corresponding to a primary complex.

Decision: Insufficient evidence to reach a decision.

448

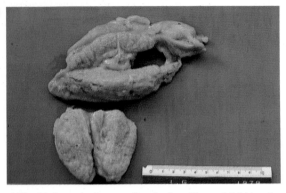

448 Tuberculosis – mediastinal and bronchial lymph node: cattle Calcified caseous tuberculosis. Reticulated caseation. A careful search for lesions in other organs or tissues was negative.

Decision: Approval, with elimination of the heart and lungs.

449

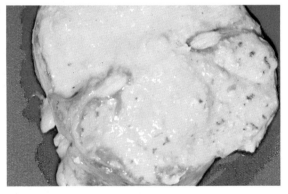

449 Caseous tuberculosis – retropharyngeal lymph nodes: cattle Caseous tuberculosis with haemorrhagic foci and softening of the caseum.

Differential diagnosis: Purulent lymphadenitis.

Decision: Total condemnation.

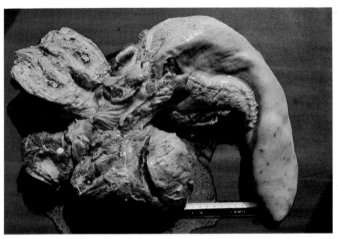

450 Tuberculosis – retropharyngeal lymph nodes: cattle The lymph nodes were enlarged and the parenchyma of one was totally replaced by caseous matter with calcified areas, which explains the stasis of the lymph. The other lymph node showed lesions corresponding to a breakdown of body resistance.

Differential diagnosis: Purulent lymphadenitis; Cysts.

Decision: Total condemnation.

451 Tuberculosis – mediastinal lymph node: cattle The lymph node was severely congested and presented large nodules of calcified caseous tuberculosis.

Decision: Insufficient material to reach a decision.

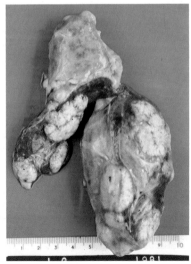

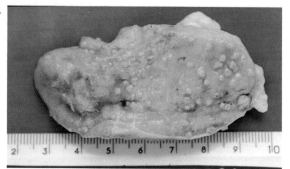

452 Tuberculosis – mediastinal lymph node: cattle
Multiple calcified caseous nodules present in this
enlarged and congested lymph node of lardaceous
appearance.

Decision: Insufficient material to reach a decision.

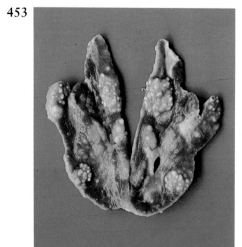

**453 Tuberculosis – lumbar lymph
node: cattle** The calcified caseous
nodules were arranged within the
lymph node in agglomerates with
more or less well-defined limits.

Decision: Insufficient material to
reach a decision.

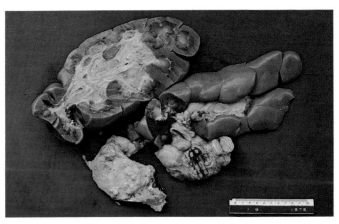

454 Tuberculosis – lumbar and renal lymph nodes: cattle
Caseous tuberculosis with softening of the caseum in one of the
lymph nodes, together with breakdown lesions.

Decision: Total condemnation.

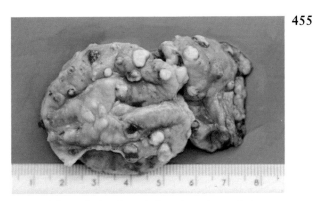

455 Tuberculosis – hepatic lymph node: cattle
Nodules of calcified caseous tuberculosis surrounded by
a congestive haemorrhagic reaction.

Decision: Insufficient elements to apply a correct
decision.

456

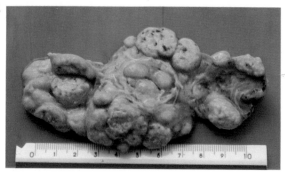

456   Tuberculosis (breakdown of body resistance) –
mesenteric lymph node: cattle   Calcified caseous
nodules, of different ages and showing haemorrhagic
foci, surrounded by fibrous tissue. The lymph node had
a bosselated appearance due to the localization of the
nodules in the cortex.

Decision: Total condemnation.

457

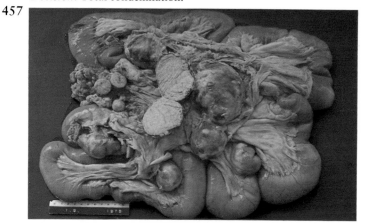

457   Tuberculosis – mesenteric lymph nodes: cattle   Calcified
caseous lesions. The cut surface of the lymph node on the left
showed stellate caseation.

Decision: Insufficient material to reach a decision.

458 Tuberculosis – pancreaticoduodenal lymph nodes: cattle The pancreaticoduodenal lymph nodes were affected by calcified caseous tuberculosis, although no tuberculous lesions were found in the pancreas. The tuberculous lesion could have been located in the duodenum; confirmation was not possible.

Decision: Approval, if no other lesions are found, with elimination of the pancreas and the intestine.

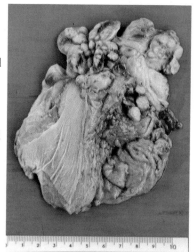

458

459 Caseous tuberculosis (breakdown form) – bronchial lymph node: cattle The centre of the organ showed numerous small tubercles, indicating the presence of microorganisms in the circulatory system.

Decision: Total condemnation.

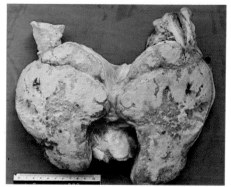

459

460

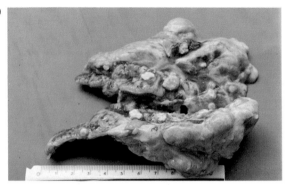

460 Tuberculosis – mediastinal lymph node: cattle
The nodules of calcified caseous tuberculosis, which were surrounded by fibrous tissue, caused partial retraction of the parenchyma and the irregularly bosselated surface of the organ.

Decision: Insufficient elements to reach a decision.

461

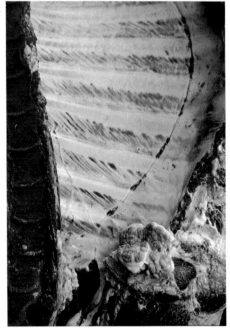

461 Tuberculosis – anterior sternal lymph node: cattle The lymph node was enlarged. The lymphoid tissue showed areas of yellow caseous necrosis, slightly prominent due to the compression of the surrounding fibrous tissue. No lesions were found in other organs and tissues drained by the lymph node.

Differential diagnosis: Actinobacillosis; Neoplasia.

Decision: Approval with elimination of the affected lymph node.

462 Nodules of caseous calcified tuberculosis – retropharyngeal lymph node: cattle Several prominent nodules are surrounded by a congestive halo. Their centres were depressed showing calcified caseum. This type of tuberculous lesion, confirmed by histopathological examination, is not typical. No lesions were found in other organs and tissues.

Decision: Approval with elimination of the head and tongue.

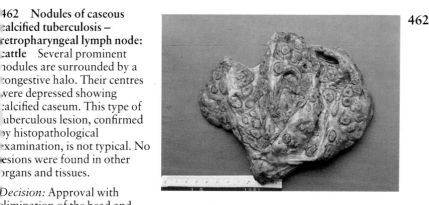

462

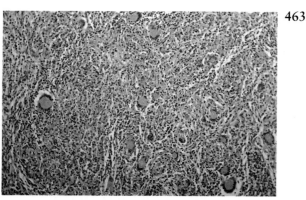

463

463 Tuberculosis – lymph node: cattle Microscopic examination of **462** revealed many epithelioid cells, Langhans' cells and lymphocytes. H. & E.

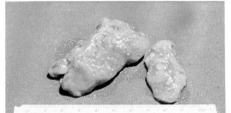

464 Tuberculosis – hepatic and mediastinal lymph nodes: horse Calcified caseous tubercles throughout the lymph nodes. No lesions were found in other organs and tissues.

Decision: Total condemnation.

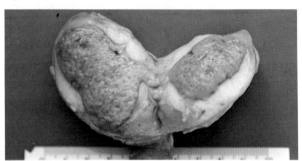

465 Actinobacillosis – retropharyngeal lymph node: cattle Incision revealed a prominent broadbean-like structure, showing whitish-yellow dots, which was totally replacing the lymphoid tissue. On compression, the organ produced a homogeneous pale yellow pus from several points.

Differential diagnosis: Tuberculosis; Metastasis from neoplasia.

Decision: Approval, with elimination of the head and tongue.

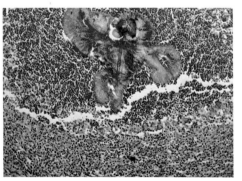

466 Actinobacillosis – lymph node: cattle Microphotograph of the lymph node shown in 465. In the centre of a microabscess a colony can be seen, with its peripheral 'clubs', already undergoing regressive changes. H. & E.

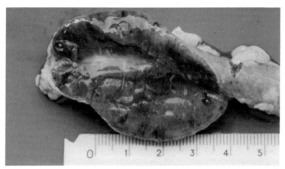

467 Linguatuliasis – mesenteric lymph node: cattle
In the cut surface there are congestive haemorrhagic lesions resulting from migrations of larvae of *Linguatula serrata*.

Decision: Approval with elimination of the intestine.

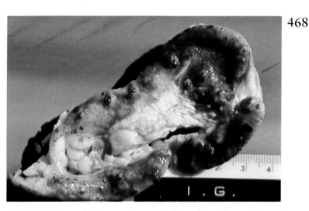

468 Linguatuliasis – mesenteric lymph node: cattle
Congestive haemorrhagic nodules formed around nymphs of *Linguatula serrata*: a more advanced stage of the lesions in **467**.

Differential diagnosis: Non-specific lymphadenitis; Metastasis from neoplasia.

Decision: Approval with elimination of the intestine.

469

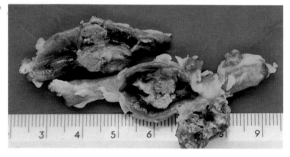

469   Linguatuliasis – mesenteric lymph node: cattle
These yellowish-green calcified necrotic lesions, encrusted on the lymph node but easily removable, resulted from the destruction of migrating larvae of *Linguatula serrata.*

Differential diagnosis: Tuberculosis.

Decision: Approval with elimination of the intestine.

470

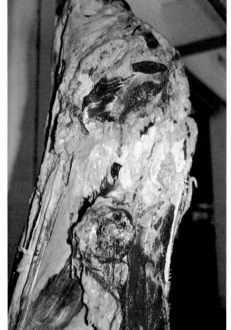

470   Carcinoma, metastasis – iliac lymph node: cattle   The lymph node was considerably enlarged due to large metastasis of a carcinoma.

Differential diagnosis: Non-specific lymphadenitis.

Decision: Total condemnation.

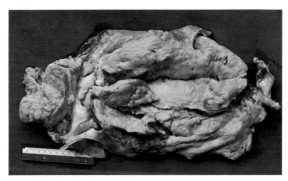

471 Carcinoma, metastasis – mediastinal and bronchial lymph nodes: cattle Numerous metastases from a carcinoma could be identified.

Differential diagnosis: Actinobacillosis; Non-specific lymphadenitis.

Decision: Total condemnation.

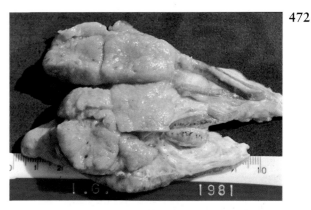

472 Carcinoma, metastasis – mediastinal lymph node: cattle

Differential diagnosis: Actinobacillosis.

Decision: Total condemnation.

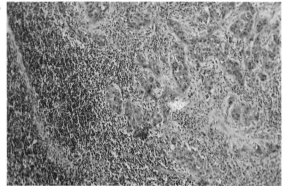

473 Epithelioma, metastasis – lymph node: cattle
The lymphoid tissue was invaded by strands of
immature epithelial cells, resulting from metastatic
growth of an epithelioma. H. & E.

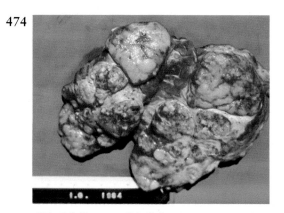

**474 Malignant epithelial tumour, metastasis –
parotid lymph node: cattle** The cut surface
showed a variety of lardaceous metastatic nodules
of a malignant epithelial tumour.

Decision: Total condemnation.

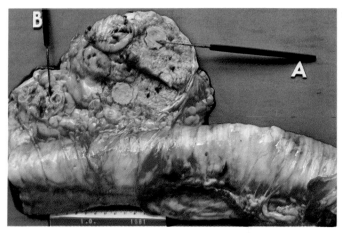

475   Epithelioma, metastasis – cervical lymph nodes: cattle
The various well-defined nodules appear either lardaceous, moist,
more-or-less haemorrhagic or even caseous, looking dry and
yellow. A and B: areas sampled for histopathological
examination.

Decision: Total condemnation.

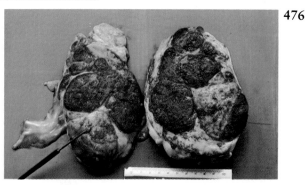

476   Epithelioma, metastasis – iliac lymph node: cattle
The enlarged lymph node showed a heterogeneous
appearance, due to the growth of several metastases of
an epithelioma, clearly individualized due to their well-
defined limits.

Decision: Total condemnation.

477

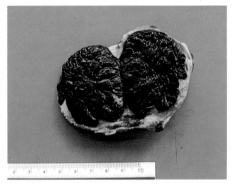

477 Melanotic sarcoma, metastasis – iliac lymph node: horse The lymphoid tissue has been replaced by a soft black tissue, which was shiny and slightly prominent.

Decision: Total condemnation.

478

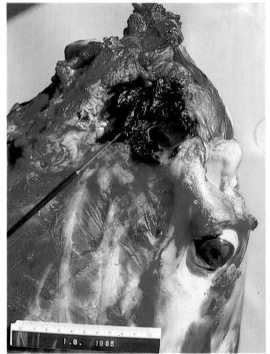

478 Malignant melanoma – parotid lymph node: horse Under the incision in the external ear a shiny black melanogenic tumour has developed from the lymph node.

Differential diagnosis: Haematoma.

Decision: Total condemnation.

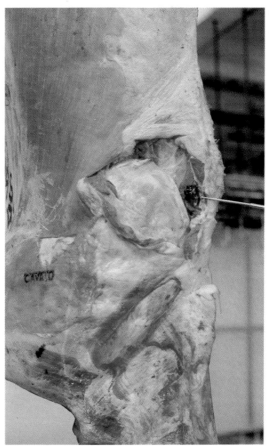

479   Malignant melanoma – subrhomboideus lymph node: horse   The shiny black subrhomboideus lymph node contains a malignant melanoma with multiple foci.

Differential diagnosis: Haematoma.

Decision: Total condemnation.

480

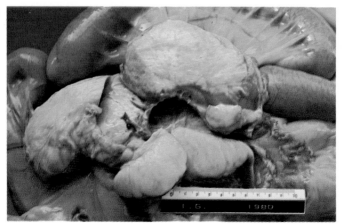

480 Undifferentiated cell sarcoma – mesenteric lymph node: cattle The cut surface of this enlarged lymph node appears solid, lardaceous, yellow, shiny and of soft consistency.

Differential diagnosis: Tuberculous lymphadenitis.

Decision: Total condemnation.

481

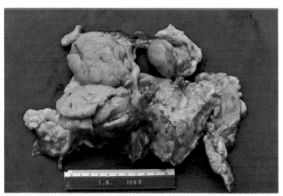

481 Undifferentiated cell sarcoma – iliac lymph node: cattle The considerably enlarged lymph nodes are yellow with a lardaceous appearance.

Differential diagnosis: Leukosis; Lymphadenitis.

Decision: Total condemnation.

482 Hypertrophy – superficial cervical lymph node: cattle
Considerable hypertrophy of the superficial cervical lymph node in an 8-year-old animal.

Hypothetical diagnosis: Leukosis; Lymphadenitis.

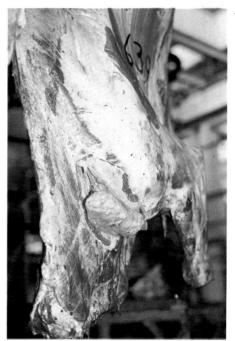

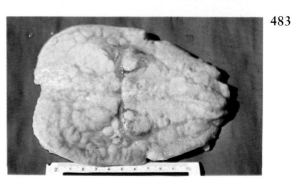

483 Lymphocytic leukosis – superficial cervical lymph node: cattle Incision of **482** reveals a yellow, soft and friable cut surface, suggesting a neoplastic process.

Decision: Total condemnation.

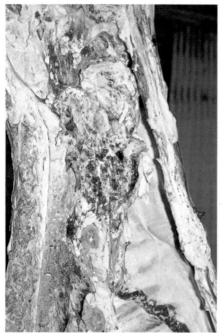

484 Lymphoblastic leukosis – infralumbar tumour: cattle A large tumefaction in the lumbosacral region. The neoplastic tissue was lardaceous, friable, not well-defined and showed multiple haemorrhages.

Decision: Total condemnation.

485 Lymphosarcoma – mediastinal and pancreatic lymph nodes: sheep The lymph nodes were enlarged and their cut surfaces shiny, yellow and friable. Undifferentiated cell lymphosarcoma. The bronchial lymph node showed areas of necrosis.

Differential diagnosis: Non-specific lymphadenitis.

Decision: Total condemnation.

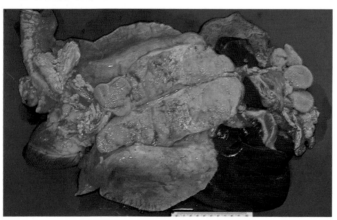

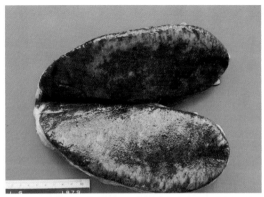

486 Lymphosarcoma – superficial cervical lymph node: cattle The lymph node was hypertrophic and the incision revealed extensive haemorrhages in the medulla and a tumoral appearance of the cortex, which was raised above the cut surface.

Decision: Total condemnation.

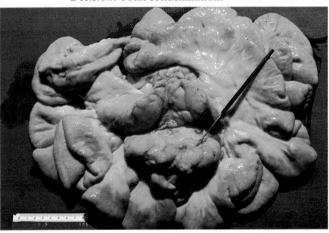

487 Lymphosarcoma – mesenteric lymph nodes: cattle The lymph nodes were markedly enlarged and at incision showed an encephaloid tissue, very soft, and with a few haemorrhagic foci.

Decision: Total condemnation.

488

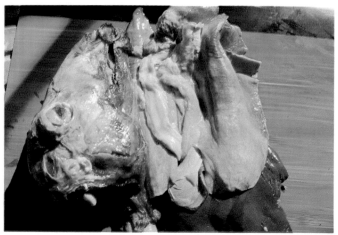

488 Lymphosarcoma – lymph nodes: sheep The lymph nodes of the head (the parotid node can be seen in the picture) and the mediastinal nodes were enlarged and showed a homogeneous, shiny and moist cut surface.

Differential diagnosis: Non-specific lymphadenitis.

Decision: Total condemnation.

489

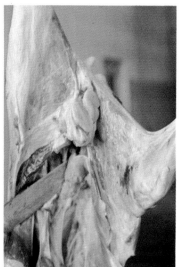

489 Lymphosarcoma – superficial inguinal and iliac lymph nodes: sheep The same animal as **488**.

Decision: Total condemnation.
Note: All lymph nodes examined, in the carcase and in the viscera, were equally involved.

490 Malignant lymphoma – carcase: sheep Subcutaneous nodules of lardaceous appearance and well-defined limits in the costal region. Their structure was similar to lymph nodes affected by leukosis.

Differential diagnosis: Lipoma; inflammatory lesions due to branding.

Decision: Total condemnation.

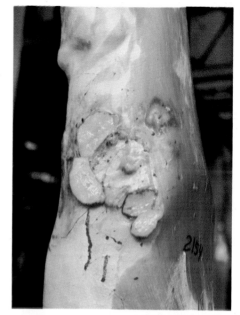

491 Prolymphocytic lymphosarcoma – superficial cervical lymph node: cattle Gross enlargement of the lymph node, whose section showed a yellowish lardaceous friable tissue, with extensive haemorrhages and necrotic foci.

Differential diagnosis: Non-specific lymphadenitis.

Decision: Total condemnation.

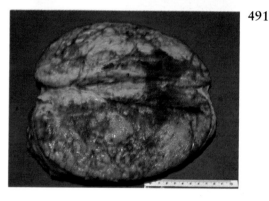

492

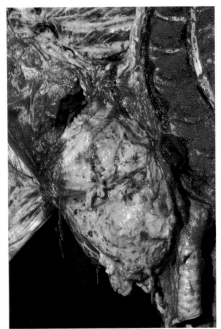

492 Lymphoblastic lymphosarcoma – lymph node: cattle
A neoplasia developed from the lymph nodes at the entrance to the chest. The tissue was encephaloid and showed small focal haemorrhages, which suggested a diagnosis of lymphosarcoma.

Decision: Total condemnation.

493

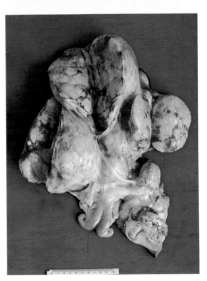

493 Lymphoblastic lymphosarcoma – lymph nodes: sheep Some normal organs of the urogenital apparatus of a ewe. Contrasting with their volume, a few pelvic lymph nodes can be seen, which were considerably hypertrophic. Their cut surface was yellow, shiny and lardaceous with a few focal haemorrhages.

Decision: Total condemnation.

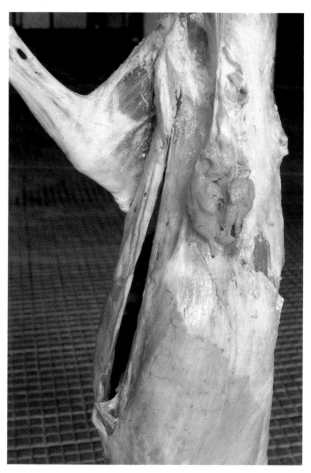

494 Lymphoblastic lymphosarcoma – carcase (flank): sheep   In the subcutaneous tissue, near the subiliac lymph node a neoplasia, the size of a fist was formed, whose macroscopical appearance resembled resting mammary tissue, although it was slightly shiny.

Decision: Total condemnation.

495

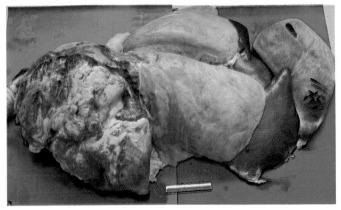

495 Plasmocytoma – viscera: horse A very large neoplasia in the cranial lobe of the left lung which was partly destroyed. The tumour also involved the heart serosa.

Differential diagnosis: Exudative pneumonia.

Decision: Total condemnation.

496

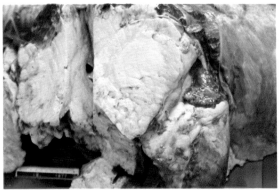

496 Plasmocytoma – viscera: horse Same case as **495**. The cut surface of this neoplasia, which developed from the pulmonary tissue, showed a whitish-yellow colour and a solid structure. The central area was paler in contrast with the pinkish peripheral region. The heart serosa was also involved.

Decision: Total condemnation.

497 Haemal nodes – carcase: sheep The haemal nodes are arranged in the lumbosacral region in a grape-like fashion. They are normal structures, frequent in ruminants, although their number in this case was abnormally high.

Differential diagnosis: Mesothelioma.

Decision: Approval with elimination of the haemal nodes.

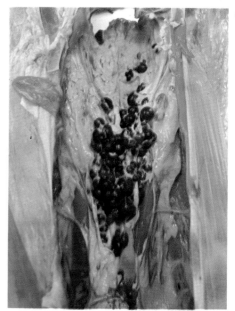

Spleen

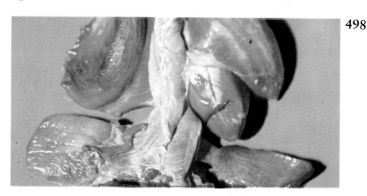

498 Accessory spleen – viscera: sheep Duplication of the spleen with abnormal localization. Both organs showed a structure close to normal, being localized just behind the diaphragm. The spleen on the left was particularly adherent to this organ.

Decision: Approval.

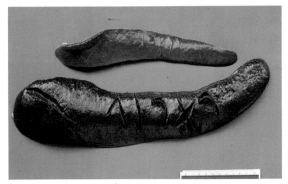

499 Congestive haemorrhagic splenitis – spleen: swine
The organ below was markedly enlarged and very dark
due to large amounts of blood it retained.

Differential diagnosis: Splenitis in erysipelas.

Decision: Approval with elimination of the spleen.

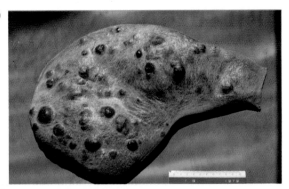

500 Multiple haematomas – spleen: horse
Numerous prominent round nodules on the surface of
the spleen. At incision they were identified as splenic
tissue particularly infiltrated with blood.

Differential diagnosis: Metastasis of a neoplasia.

Decision: Approval with elimination of the spleen.

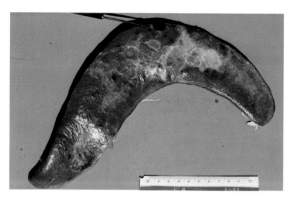

**501 Perisplenitis and focal haemorrhages – spleen:
swine** Under the capsule, small haemorrhagic foci
could be noticed. The capsule showed signs of an old
inflammatory lesion with connective tissue
organization.

Differential diagnosis: Hog cholera.

Decision: Approval with elimination of the spleen.

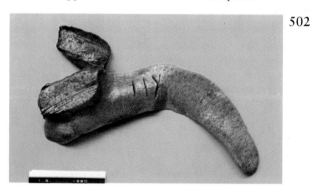

502 Necrohaemorrhagic splenitis – spleen: swine
A large ovoid tumour was identified at the surface of the
spleen. When sectioned it showed splenic tissue with
areas of necrosis and haemorrhages.

Decision: Approval with elimination of the spleen.

503

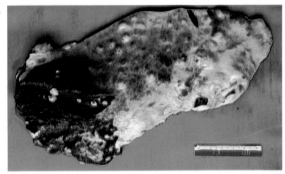

503 Purulent necrotic splenitis – spleen: cattle The capsule showed clear signs of chronic inflammation, and underneath small foci of yellow pasty pus were identified.

Bacteriology of the pus: Negative.

Differential diagnosis: Tuberculosis; Actinobacillosis or actinomycosis.

Decision: Approval, after thermal treatment, subject to the results of the laboratory examinations, with elimination of the spleen. If simultaneously embolic abscesses are found in the liver, there is total condemnation.

504

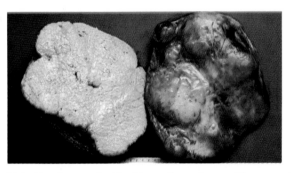

504 Focal necrotic splenitis – spleen: sheep The organ became spherical; several round nodules, prominent under the capsule were identified. They were white and appeared neoplastic. The incision showed a process of necrosis, similar to caseation, with areas of dystrophic calcification.

Differential diagnosis: Neoplasia; Tuberculosis.

Decision: Approval, subject to the results of the laboratory examination, or approval conditional to thermal treatment, with elimination of the spleen.

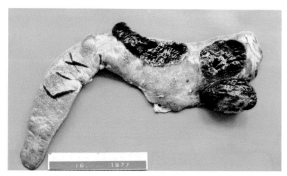

505 Necrotic splenitis – spleen: swine Under the fibrous capsule there were several tumefactions. The incision showed they were formed of highly haemorrhagic splenic tissue with some yellowish areas of necrosis.

Differential diagnosis: Neoplasia.

Decision: Approval with elimination of the spleen.

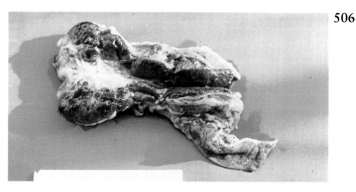

506 Chronic splenitis – spleen: swine The spleen was considerably modified showing two distinct portions: a swollen one, very consistent and hard to cut due to the development of fibrous tissue and another atrophic area with a wrinkly capsule.

Decision: Approval with elimination of the spleen.

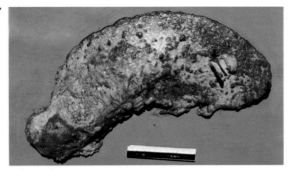

507 Tuberculosis – spleen (capsule): cattle Specific inflammatory disease affecting the serosa of the spleen. Small pink or dark-red nodules could be noticed. Incision of one of them showed abundant caseous matter. The carcase and viscera presented identical lesions due to generalization.

Differential diagnosis: Actinobacillosis; Non-specific splenitis; Neoplasia.

Decision: Total condemnation.

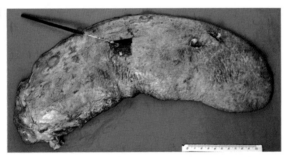

508 Tuberculosis – spleen: cattle Some of the small raised and pale areas which could be seen under the capsule were surrounded by a congestive halo. Incision revealed yellow necrotic nodules with central calcification.

Differential diagnosis: Actinobacillosis; Multiple abscesses.

Decision: Total condemnation.

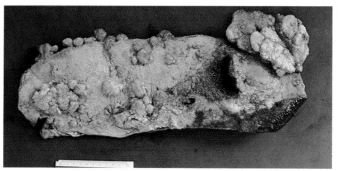

509   **Pearl disease (tuberculosis) – spleen: cattle**   A series of pinkish cauliflower-like nodules under the capsule of the spleen. Incision revealed nodules of caseous necrosis. No lesions were noticed inside the organ. The pleura and lungs presented similar lesions.

Differential diagnosis: Actinobacillosis; Non-specific granulomas; Metastasis of neoplasia.

Decision: Total condemnation.

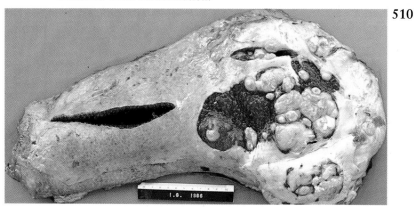

510   **Actinomycosis – spleen: cattle**   On the right side of the organ lesions of actinomycosis have developed, leading to a localized hypertrophy. The nodules shown by the incision contained a yellow-straw pus. The central area of the older nodules was transformed into a voluminous abscess, with a viscous yellow elastic pus.

Differential diagnosis: Tuberculosis; Unspecific abscesses; Necrobacillosis.

Decision: Approval, if no other lesions are found, with elimination of the spleen.

511

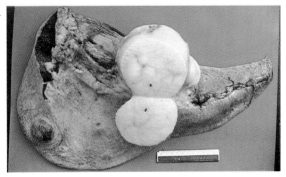

511 Lipoma and haematoma – spleen: horse The ventral surface of the spleen presented two different types of lesions. The larger one was spherical, whitish and adherent to the capsule by a broad pedicle. It corresponded to a benign neoplasia. The second was a small parenchymal bluish nodule, slightly prominent, corresponding to a small haematoma.

Decision: Approval with elimination of the spleen.

512

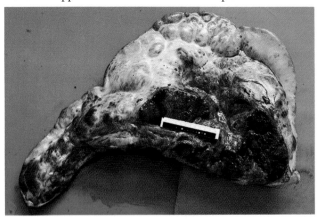

512 Spindle-cell sarcoma – spleen: horse The profile of the spleen was modified by rounded nodules, which tended to form agglomerates. The capsule was golden-yellow. The cut surface was polychromatic, with bright red and dark red areas, the latter being haemorrhagic lesions.

Decision: Total condemnation.

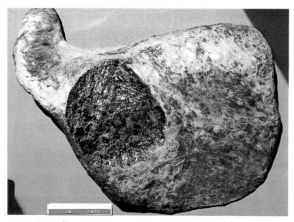

513 Spindle-cell sarcoma – spleen: horse The enlarged spleen presented in some areas of the capsule increased vascularization, sometimes assuming a star-like appearance. The parenchyma was equally abnormal, with bright red areas alternating with dark red haemorrhagic ones.

Differential diagnosis: Hyperplastic splenomegaly; Hyperaemia.

Decision: Total condemnation.

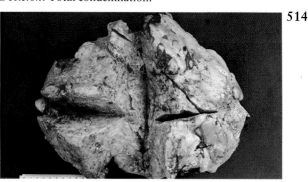

514 Fibrosarcoma – spleen: horse A malignant tumour of the connective tissue nearly destroyed the spleen. The consistency was increased and the yellowish neoplastic tissue showed multiple haemorrhages. A few portions of the capsule can be seen in the lower right side and in the upper left.

Decision: Total condemnation.

515

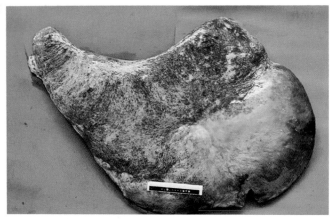

515 Sarcoma – spleen: horse The spleen was very much enlarged, particularly in the broader region, where it presented rounded margins. The golden-yellow capsule was congested, assuming a bright-red colour in some areas.

Decision: Total condemnation.

516

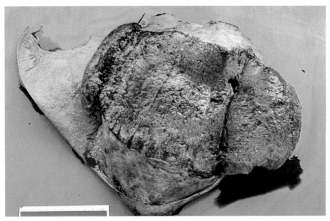

516 Fibrosarcoma – spleen: horse A large tumefaction occupied most of the spleen. Incision revealed a firm tissue, yellow-orange with a few haemorrhages.

Differential diagnosis: Haematoma.

Decision: Total condemnation.

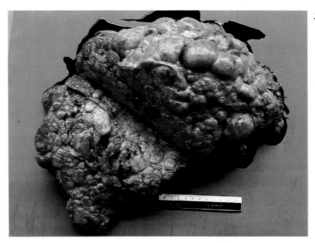

517 Fibrosarcoma – spleen: horse The spleen was totally replaced by a tumour of the connective tissue. The surface of the neoplasia was bosselated with nodules of various sizes. The tissue of the tumour was nodular, solid and pinkish.

Decision: Total condemnation.

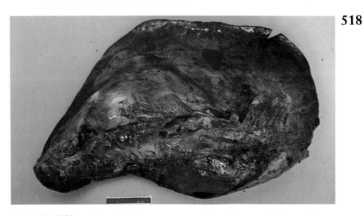

518 Undifferentiated cell sarcoma – spleen: horse The weight of this considerably enlarged spleen was 26 kg. The margins were rounded, particularly the thickened central area. The dark colour was due to the accumulation of blood within the organ.

Decision: Total condemnation.

519

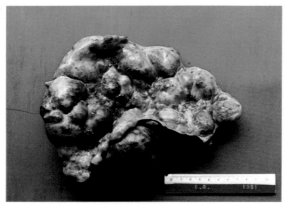

519   Undifferentiated cell sarcoma – spleen: horse
The spleen was atrophic and its morphology deeply
changed due to the development of a multinodular
neoplasia.

Decision: Total condemnation.

520

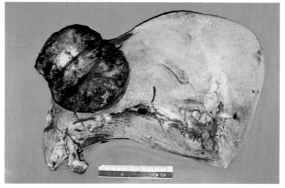

520   Undifferentiated cell sarcoma – spleen: horse   A
rounded neoplasia developed in the spleen. Incision
showed a yellowish tissue, with haemorrhages at the
periphery.

Differential diagnosis: Haematoma.

Decision: Total condemnation.

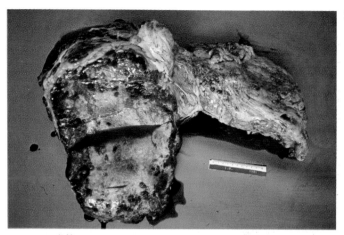

521 **Undifferentiated cell sarcoma – spleen: horse**   A very large
bosselated neoplasia, with a spherical shape 20 cm in diameter
was attached to one of the extremities, spreading diffusely in the
organ. Incision showed a yellow tissue with haemorrhages in the
periphery.

Decision: Total condemnation.

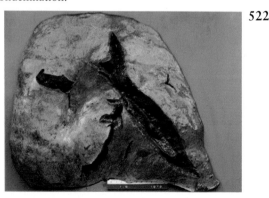

522   **Undifferentiated cell sarcoma – spleen: horse**   The spleen was
hypertrophic with rounded margins and soft consistency. Incisions revealed pale
tissue with disseminated yellow neoplastic nodules.

Differential diagnosis: Congestive haemorrhagic splenitis.

Decision: Total condemnation.

523

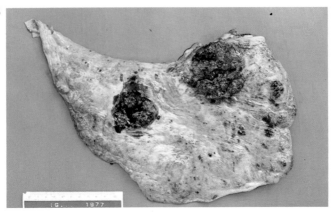

523   Undifferentiated cell sarcoma – spleen: horse   Nodules of various sizes could be seen under the capsule. Their incision showed a pink, shiny and friable tissue, amid haemorrhages of variable extent.

Decision: Total condemnation.

524

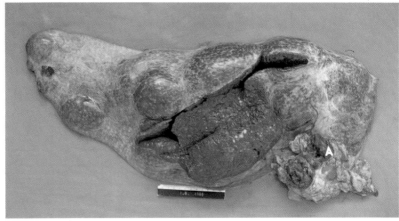

524   Undifferentiated cell sarcoma – spleen: cattle   The spleen profile was severely modified due to the existence of various nodules, several centimetres in diameter, prominent under the capsule. Incision showed a slight increased consistency, and a tumoral yellow tissue, forming small nodules, only a few millimetres in diameter.

Decision: Total condemnation.

525 Haemangiosarcoma – spleen: horse Underneath the capsule, there was a prominent, round swelling. It was firm and the colour varied from yellow in the centre to a pinkish tone at the periphery. The proximal pole of the neoplasia was dark-red due to the accumulation of blood.

Differential diagnosis: Haematoma undergoing organization.

Decision: Total condemnation.

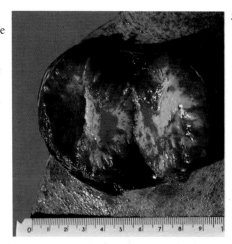

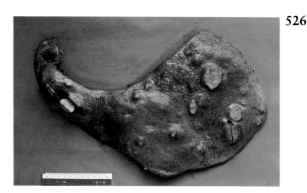

526 Carcinoma, metastasis – spleen: horse
Yellow nodules of well-defined limits and firm consistency in the spleen, surrounded by a congestive halo. The incision showed they were deeply embedded in the organ, although without being invasive.

Differential diagnosis: Non-specific granulomas; Actinobacillosis.

Decision: Total condemnation.

Thymus

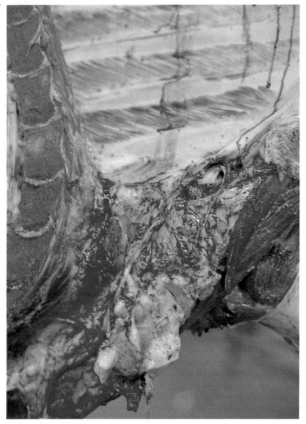

527 Thymoma – thorax and jugular groove: cattle A large voluminous tissue mass, white and firm, with multiple petechial haemorrhages, at the anterior end of the thorax and along the neck close to the jugular vein (jugular groove – *Sulcus jugularis*). The microscopical examination showed that it was formed by lymphocytes, between which was a considerable number of epithelial cells, with clear nuclei and large nucleoli.

Decision: Total condemnation.

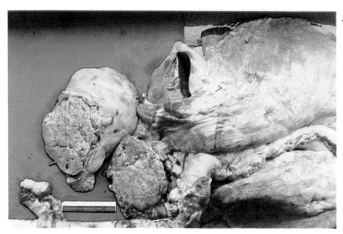

528 Thymoma – thymus: horse   In the anterior end of the thoracic cavity, close to the sternum and the cranial part of the lungs, a large encapsulated neoplasia was identified. The incision showed it was moderately firm, mostly yellow and pinkish.

Decision: Total condemnation.

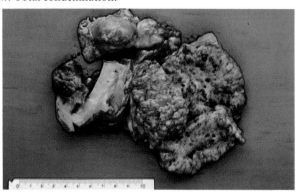

529 Epithelial thymoma – thymus: cattle   A swelling in the thoracic cavity, contiguous with the first rib and the internal thoracic artery, was surrounded by a delicate fibrous capsule. Its profile was highly irregular due to the development of several small nodules. The cut surface showed the central area occupied by fibrous tissue.

Differential diagnosis: Tuberculosis; Actinobacillosis.

Decision: Total condemnation.

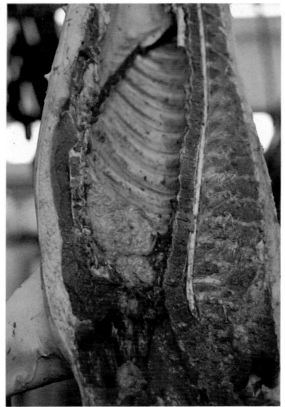

530 Thymic lymphosarcoma – thymus: swine An encephaloid-like mass of soft consistency in the ventral cranial part of the thorax, which corresponded to a thymic lymphosarcoma.

Decision: Total condemnation.

531 Thymic lymphosarcoma – thymus: horse A large swelling over the first rib, appearing like fetal lung, with small round whitish nodules.

Decision: Total condemnation.

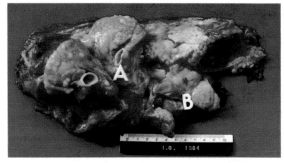

531

532 Thymic lymphosarcoma – thymus: cattle A large glandular-like swelling extended from the entrance of the chest up to the cranial part of the neck, totally occupying the jugular groove.

Decision: Total condemnation.

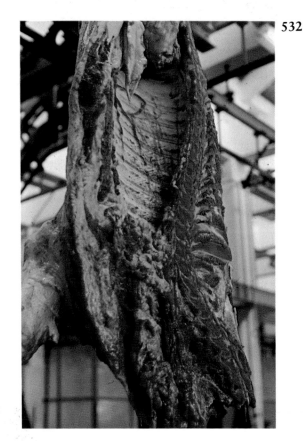

532

533

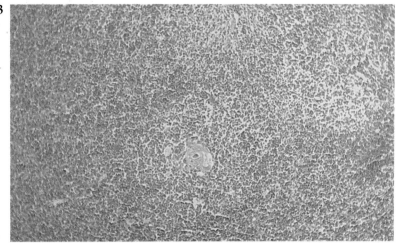

533   Thymic lymphosarcoma – thymus: cattle   The normal thymus has been almost totally replaced by neoplastic lymphoid tissue. A Hassall corpuscle can be seen in the centre of the microphotograph. H. & E.

534

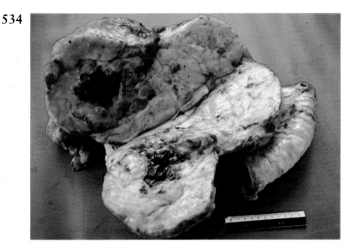

534   Thymic lymphosarcoma – thymus: cattle   A large tumefaction extended from the middle of the ventral border of the neck up to the first rib, sometimes adhering to neighbouring tissue. The section showed a shiny yellowish tissue containing a small cavity filled with clotted blood.

Decision: Total condemnation.

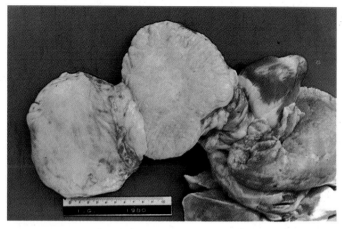

535 Thymic lymphosarcoma – thymus: sheep An encapsulated globular swelling in the thorax near the heart, related with the auricles. The section showed two different areas: a central white one surrounded by a yellowish peripheral area.

Differential diagnosis: Neurofibroma.

Decision: Total condemnation.

7: The respiratory system

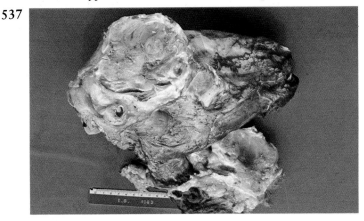

536 Fibrous polyp – nasal cavity: horse A large polyp in the nasal cavity reaching to the posterior nares.

Decision: Approval with elimination of the neoplasia.

537 Fibro-osteoma – lateral frontal sinus: sheep In the dome-shaped right frontal sinus, a mass of newly formed tissue was observed, after removal of the superficial tissues. This was white and well irrigated, although it did not have the usual appearance of malignant neoplasia.

Differential diagnosis: Malignant neoplasia.

Decision: Approval with elimination of the head.

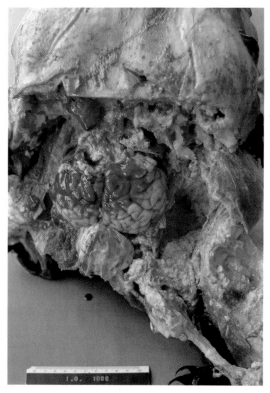

538 Empyema – occipital sinuses: cattle The left occipital sinuses were partially filled with a purulent greenish-grey matter, with granular appearance, more or less solidified.

Decision: Approval with elimination of the affected tissues.

539

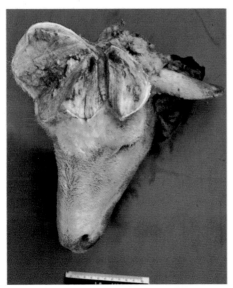

539 Squamous cell carcinoma – frontal sinus: sheep A large neoplasia, resembling a horn, originated from the frontal sinus totally invading the cavity. The incision showed it had a lardaceous appearance and was infected centrally.

Decision: Total condemnation.

540

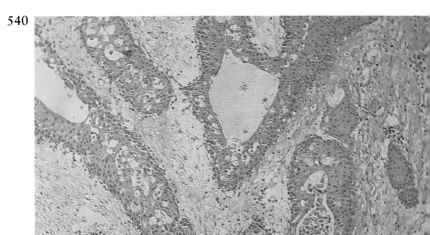

540 Squamous cell carcinoma – frontal sinus: sheep A carcinoma, arising from the respiratory epithelium covering the sinus, with the morphology of a squamous cell carcinoma. H. & E.

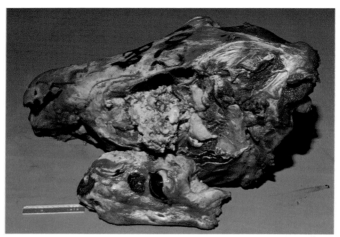

541 Squamous cell carcinoma and empyema – upper jaw (sinus): horse On the left paranasal sinus a pinkish, shiny and soft neoplasia developed, occupying part of the cavities. The sinuses were filled with yellowish-green purulent matter, more or less solidified.

Differential diagnosis: Glanders.

Decision: Total condemnation.

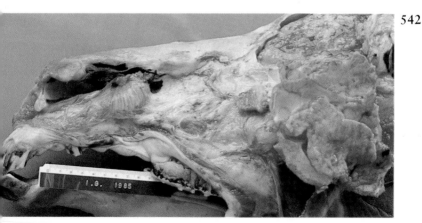

42 Adenocarcinoma – nasal sinuses: horse A neoplasia in the paranasal nuses, deforming the nasal bones. The exploratory incision showed a tissue with roplastic characteristics.

ecision: Total condemnation.

543

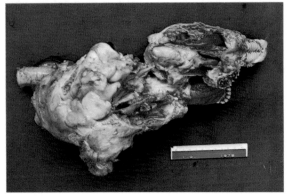

543 Carcinoma of the ethmoid – paranasal sinuses: sheep A particularly marked exophthalmus of the left eye justified a detailed post-mortem examination of the head. The mandibular bone was sectioned near the mandibular articulation and the upper frontal part of the head was removed uncovering a multilobated lardaceous neoplasia, whitish-yellow, located in the ethmoid area.

Decision: Total condemnation.

544

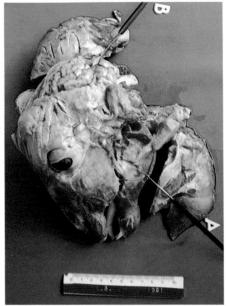

544 Osteosarcoma – maxillary sinus: goat The head showed an abnormal rounded shape. A compac tissue had invaded the superior maxillary sinus and a considerable area of the left lower jaw (A). The neoplasia had the appearance of muscle with small calcified foci. B slight brain oedema.

Decision: Total condemnation.

**5 Peripharyngeal – laryngeal
…ema: cattle** At the back of the
…gue and mouth an abundant
…owish serogelatinous oedema was
…ntified. The removal of the tongue
…nulated the drainage of most of
…fluid of the oedema, and the
…ues reassumed their normal
…pearance.

…cision: Approval with elimination
…he head and tongue.

…is type of oedema is frequently
…nd in badly-transported cattle,
…ally in the hold of a ship, where,
…rt from the high temperature, the
…mals are permanently subjected to
…tant vapours due to accumulation
…faeces and urine. This type of
…lema is also frequently noticed in
…es of pasteurellosis; in allergic
…ctions; due to the action of foreign
…dies and to surrounding passive
…igestion. Any decision has to take
…o consideration the
…iopathogenicity of the process and
…repercussion in the meat.

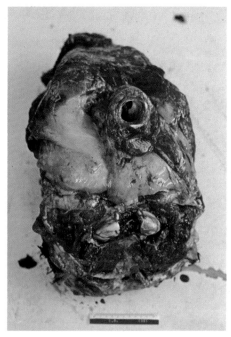

**5 Strangles –
…ilaryngeal tissues:**
…rse Necropurulent
…ammatory reaction of
…perilaryngeal tissues
…l swelling of the
…ional lymph nodes
…rulent adenitis). The
…mal was well fed,
…rretic and showed no
…ns of general systemic
…ction.

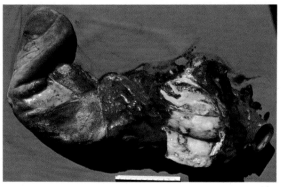

…cteriological examination: This showed *Streptococcus equi.*

…fferential diagnosis: Glanders; Angina.

…cision: Approval with elimination of the head and tongue.

547

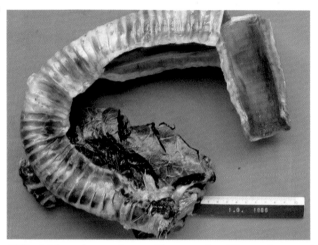

547   Melanosis – trachea and lung: cattle   The trachea was black, particularly between the cartilaginous rings, near the bifurcation. A fragment of the lung, which was jointly removed, showed similar lesions. This pigmentation can also be seen through the tracheal mucosa. The changes had affected other organs.

Decision: Total condemnation.

548

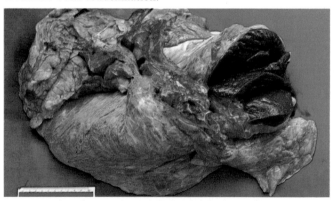

548   Abnormal localization of a fragment of liver-lung: cattle A dark red round mass, surrounded by a fibrous capsule in the right diaphragmatic lobe. Incision revealed similar characteristics to normal liver, which was confirmed by histopathological examination. A fibrous scar was present in the diaphragm.

Differential diagnosis: Haematoma; Neoplasia.

Decision: Approval with elimination of the ectopic liver fragment.

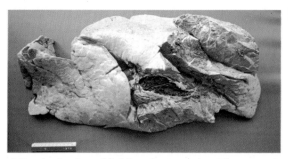

549 Aspiration of fodder – lung: cattle The incision of the emphysematous lungs showed that all bronchi were filled with vegetable particles. The accident was due to regurgitation of the rumen content, followed by aspiration, a situation that frequently occurs during slaughter.

Decision: Approval with elimination of the lungs.

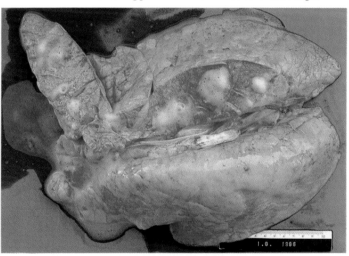

550 Scalding water aspiration – lung: swine The lungs were hypertrophic due to alveolar emphysema, which was formed during the agony stage. The bronchi and bronchioles were filled with foam mixed with fluid, resulting from inhalation of water during scalding.

Differential diagnosis: Acute pulmonary oedema.

Decision: Approval with elimination of the lungs.

551

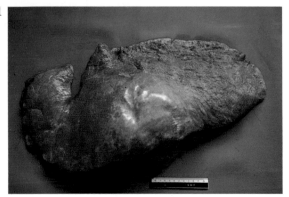

551 Collapse – lung: horse Most of the lung had collapsed, with compensatory emphysema of the remaining area. There was a clear difference in colour between both parts of the lung, corresponding to each type of lesion.

Differential diagnosis: Atelectasis.

Decision: Approval with elimination of the lungs.

552

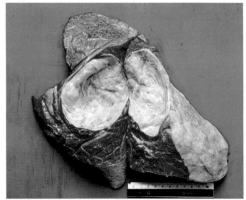

552 Cyst containing gas – lung: cattle Within the lung, under the pleura, the tissue bulged abnormally. Incision revealed a cyst with a fibrous wall, containing an uncharacteristic gas.

Differential diagnosis: Bronchiectasis.

Decision: Approval with elimination of the affected lung.

553 Supranumerary lobe – lung: sheep
A spherical mass 6 cm in diameter in the cranial lobe, attached by a pedicle of dense pulmonary tissue. It had the consistency of an emphysema and it crepitated intensely when sectioned due to the excessive accumulation of air in the alveoli.

Differential diagnosis: Neoplasia.

Decision: Approval with elimination of the supranumerary lobe.

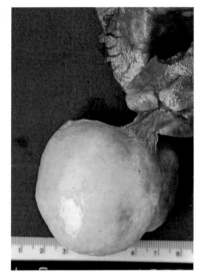

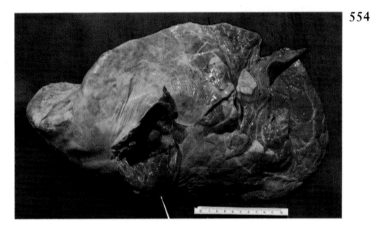

554 Emphysema – lung: cattle   The lung, thickened by visceral pleura presented a small swollen area. The incision showed it was an accumulation of odourless gas, with no particular characteristics, contained within a cavity limited by parenchyma with atelectasis.

Differential diagnosis: Bronchiectasis; Tuberculous cavern.

Decision: Approval, with elimination of the affected tissues.

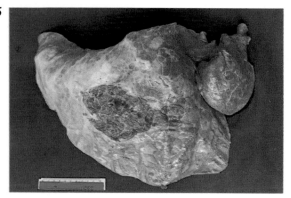

555 **Emphysema – lung: cattle**   Lobulation was due to an interstitial emphysema, which could be clearly seen under the pleura and deep within the organ.

Decision: Approval with elimination of the lung.

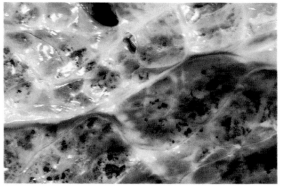

556 **Melanosis (congenital) – lung: cattle**   Small black patches of variable shape at the surface of a calf's lung, due to the deposition of melanotic pigment.

Differential diagnosis: Haemorrhages (petechial); Metastasis of a neoplasia.

Decision: Approval with elimination of the lungs.

557   Melanosis (congenital) – lung: cattle   Small black areas disseminated through the lungs. There were identical patches in the mediastinal and bronchial lymph nodes.

Differential diagnosis: Anthracosis; Metastasis of neoplasia; Haemorrhages.

Decision: Total condemnation due to the involvement of the lymph nodes.
Several authors advise total condemnation if it is impossible to remove completely the affected tissues and organs.

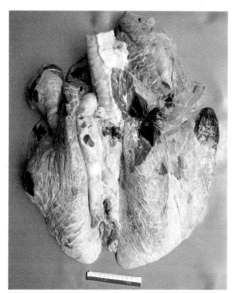

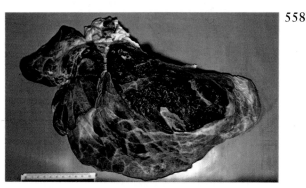

558   Diffuse melanosis – lung: cattle   This calf's lung was completely infiltrated by melanin pigment. Identical lesions were seen in the heart, kidneys and liver of the same animal.

Differential diagnosis: Anthracosis.

Decision: Total condemnation due to generalization of the process.

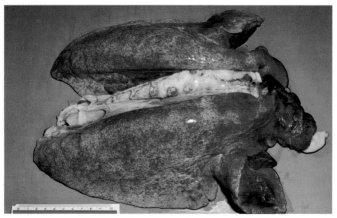

559 Agonal aspiration of blood – lung: swine The lung was totally collapsed and under the pleura were countless small haemorrhages. This lesion is frequent due to agonal aspiration of the scalding water.

Differential diagnosis: Venous hyperaemia; Septic haemorrhages.

Decision: Approval with elimination of the lungs.
Note: Similar lesions may occur in the lungs of swine and sheep stunned by a deficient electrical current voltage.

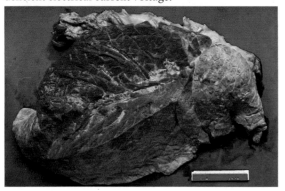

560 Active hyperaemia – lung: cattle Under the pleura, extensive areas of irregular profile and marked pink colour were seen. The incision revealed a deep red parenchyma due to active congestion of the capillaries, corresponding to the initial stage of an inflammatory reaction.

Differential diagnosis: Passive hyperaemia; Agonal aspiration of blood.

Decision: Approval subject to the results of the laboratory examinations, with elimination of the lungs.

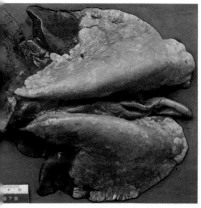 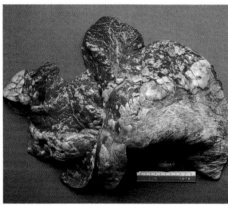

561 Exudative pneumonia – lung: sheep The cranial lobes and the anterior part of the diaphragmatic lobe showed a red colour and increased consistency similar to the liver. The affected parts, when put in water, sank and their incision revealed an absence of crepitation. The described characteristics correspond to the red consolidation (hepatization) stage of the lobar pneumonia.

Decision: Total condemnation.
Alternatively, approval after thermal treatment, with elimination of thoracic viscera, if the laboratory examination of meat and abdominal viscera is negative. If economically feasible, taking into account the variety of lesions which may be present in pneumonia, the following inspection criteria for post-mortem examination should be considered:
(a) Total condemnation: in cases of necrotic pneumonia, or any form of acute pneumonia.
(b) Approval conditional to thermal treatment, subject to the results of the laboratory examinations, with elimination of the lungs and pleuras:
   (i) in cases of subacute pneumonia in any slaughter animal;
   (ii) in cases of aspiration pneumonia.
(c) Approval in cases of catarrhal pneumonia with no suspicion of bacteraemia.

562 Exudative pneumonia – lung: cattle Lesions of red consolidation were noted in the cranial lobes extending to other lobes. The unaffected lobes were distended due to abnormal accumulation of air.

Decision: Total condemnation.
Alternatively, the decision could be approval, after heat treatment, and provided that laboratory results are negative.

563

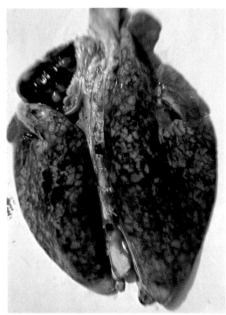

563 Acute oedema (African swine fever) – lung: swine This enlarged lung did not collapse after the opening of the thoracic cavity, as a consequence of the severe oedema affecting the alveoli, the interlobula and the interlobar tissue. The parenchyma was dark-red due to extensive haemorrhages of the superficial capillaries.

Differential diagnosis: Oedema due to chronic passive congestion (cardiac oedema); Aspiration of scalding water.

Decision: Total condemnation.

564

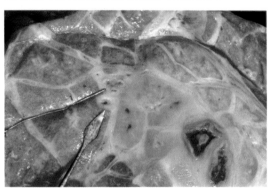

564 Chronic interstitial pneumonia – lung: cattle Foci of pneumonia involved several adjacent lobules whose colour varied from yellowish to pink or red, separated by fibrous septa, which showed some oedema due to stasis of the lymph.

Bacteriological examination: This showed *Pasteurella multocida*.

Differential diagnosis: Contagious bovine pleuropneumonia.

Decision: Approval with elimination of the lungs.

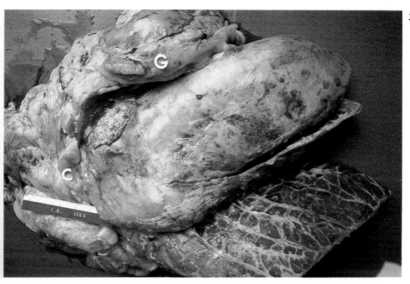

565 Contagious bovine pleuropneumonia – lung: cattle   The diaphragmatic lobe was markedly hypertrophic and did not collapse on opening the thoracic cavity. The consistency was increased (hepatization) and the cut surface exuded abundant yellow fluid (pleuropneumonic lymph).
The cut surface of the affected lobe showed a particularly sharp lobular division due to the perilobular oedema. C and G: lymph nodes.

Differential diagnosis: Interstitial emphysema; Aspiration pneumonia; Interstitial pneumonia.

Decision: Approval with elimination of the thoracic viscera and the costal pleura. The decision 'approval for human consumption with distribution restricted to limited areas' should be considered, if an outbreak of a dangerous contagious disease such as bovine pleuropneumonia occurs in some areas.

566

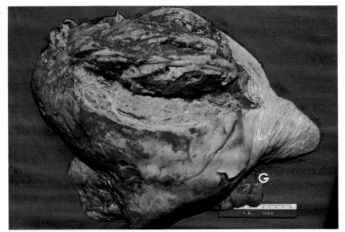

566 Contagious bovine pleuropneumonia (sequestrum) – lung: cattle The palpation of the diaphragmatic lobe revealed a more consistent part, corresponding to an increase in the pleural thickness. Incision revealed an area of necrosis surrounded by a fibrous capsule, which clearly separates it from the normal neighbouring tissues. G: lymph node.

Differential diagnosis: Tuberculosis; Actinobacillosis; Abscess; Aspiration pneumonia.

Decision: Approval with elimination of the thoracic viscera and costal pleura.

567

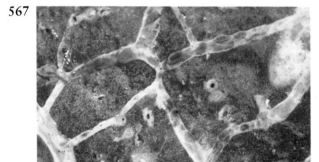

567 Contagious bovine pleuropneumonia – lung: cattle Increased density of the pulmonary parenchyma can be clearly seen. The lobules are separated by connective tissue septa, thickened due to an oedema caused by multiple thrombosis of the lymph vessels.

568   Contagious bovine pleuropneumonia (perivascular foci of organized inflammatory tissue) lung: cattle   Magnification of an affected lung showing perivascular foci of organized inflammatory tissue in the interlobular tissue and some foci around intralobular bronchi. Such foci are considered pathognomonic of this disease.

Differential diagnosis: Chronic interstitial pneumonia.

Decision: Approval with elimination of the thoracic viscera and costal pleura. In cases of bovine pleuropneumonia, total condemnation is recommended:
a) When the meat is from feverish animals.
b) When the meat shows signs of general systemic reaction.
c) When the meat reveals signs of acute disease.
d) If the meat is from juveniles.
e) If polyarthritis, degeneration of parenchymatous organs or marked emaciation are present.

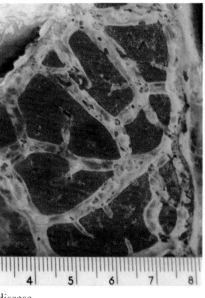

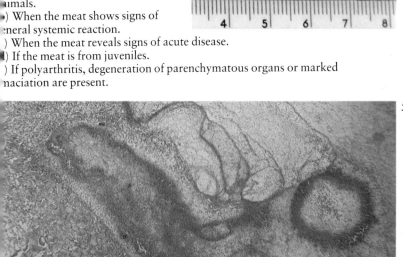

569   Contagious bovine pleuropneumonia. Perivascular foci of organized inflammatory tissue – lung: cattle   In a highly dilated interlobular septum due to stasis of the lymph, perivascular foci of organized inflammatory tissue can be seen. This is considered a decisive element for the microscopical diagnosis of the disease. H. & E.

570

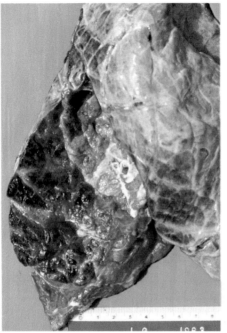

570 Haemorrhagic bronchopneumonia – lung: cattle
The section of the lung showed a dark areas, similar to anthracosis melanosis, but in fact correspond to a bronchopneumonia in which haemorrhages were the predomin lesions.

Differential diagnosis: Melanosis (congenital); Anthracosis.

Decision: Approval, with elimina of the lungs, subject to the results laboratory examinations.

571 Fibrinous purulent bronchopneumonia – lung: cattle
large area in the lungs was invade by a fibrinous-purulent inflamma reaction, which assumed an acina disposition, frequent in pulmonar diseases caused by *Pasteurella* sp.

Differential diagnosis: Tumour metastasis.

571

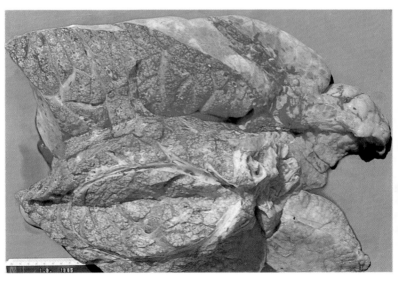

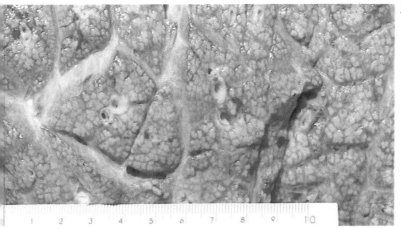

572 Fibrinous purulent bronchopneumonia (macrophotograph) – lung: cattle
Bronchopneumonia. Detail of 571.

Decision: Total condemnation or conditionally approved, with elimination of the lungs, provided thermal treatment is applied and if the bacteriological examination of the carcase and abdominal viscera is negative.

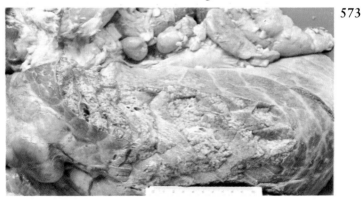

573 Purulent bronchopneumonia – lung: cattle The diaphragmatic lobe was affected by a purulent bronchopneumonia the lesions of which frequently assumed a clover-like feature, common in cases of *Pasteurella* sp. infection, which can be mistaken for tuberculous lesions (acinar form). The lymph nodes were reactive but the lesions did not suggest a tuberculous nature.

Differential diagnosis: Acinar tuberculosis.

Decision: Total condemnation.

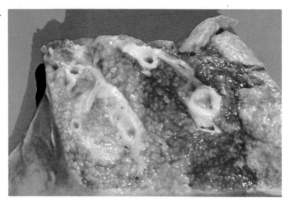

574 Purulent bronchopneumonia – lung: sheep
Magnification of a lung showing extensive lesions of
purulent bronchopneumonia as well as older lesions of
chronic bronchitis. The thickened walls of the bronchi
contained inflammatory exudate. The lesions are
classically clover-like, relatively heterogeneous with
marked congestive lesions in the central area.

Decision: Total condemnation.

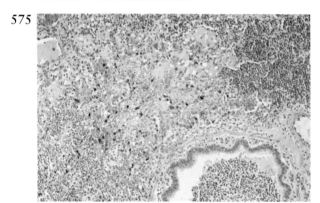

575 Purulent bronchopneumonia – lung: cattle
Lesions of alveolitis in different stages of evolution and
the bronchioli partially filled with a cellular exudate.
H. & E.

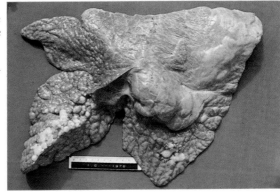

576 Suppurative pneumonia – lung: cattle
The cranial lobes and the anterior part of the diaphragmatic lobe were showing multiple miliary abscesses containing yellowish pus, corresponding to lesions of suppurative alveolitis or bronchiolitis. Emphysema was noticeable in the caudal part of the diaphragmatic lobe.

Bacteriology of the regional lymph nodes: This showed *Pasteurella multocida.*

Decision: Total condemnation.

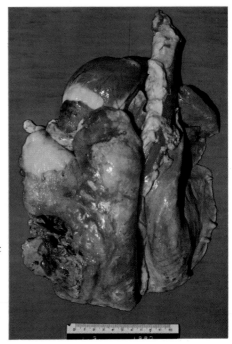

577 Suppurative pneumonia – lung: sheep The cardiac and diaphragmatic lobes of the left lung presented distinctive types of inflammatory reactions. The cardiac lobe showed lesions of pneumonia with fibrinous pleuritis and the diaphragmatic lobe an extensive necropurulent lesion with loss of tissue.

Decision: Total condemnation.

578

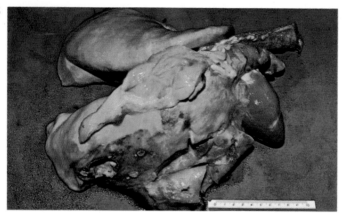

578 Necrotic gangrenous abscesses – lung: sheep A few dark areas were noticed at the surface of the lung. They were abscesses with a dark necrotic wall, containing yellowish pus in an area of inflammatory tissue. The mediastinal and bronchial lymph nodes were considerably hypertrophic and moist, as a reaction to the necrotic process.

Decision: Total condemnation.

579

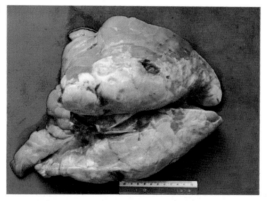

579 Enzootic pneumonia – lung: swine The affected areas of the lung were pinkish, moist and particularly friable, with the characteristics of the initial stage of enzootic pneumonia. Simultaneously compensatory emphysema was noticed in the dorsal part of the diaphragmatic lobe.

Decision: Approval conditional to thermal treatment, with elimination of the lungs and heart.
Some authors recommend approval, subject to the laboratory results, if there is a suspicion of bacteraemia, with elimination of the lungs, heart and parietal pleura.

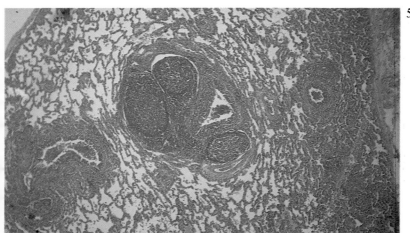

580 Enzootic pneumonia – lung: swine Large peribronchial and peribronchiolar accumulations of lymphoid cells can be seen, which compress and reduce the lumen of the bronchial tree. The parenchyma shows discrete lesions of interstitial pneumonia. H. & E.

581 Interstitial pneumonia – lungs: sheep At the opening of the thorax the lungs did not retract. The semi-elastic consistency was similar to sponge rubber with a brownish-grey colour. When cut, small rounded nodules, lardaceous, could be seen, corresponding to areas of hyperplastic lymphoid tissue in a case of progressive interstitial pneumonia.

Differential diagnosis: anthracosis.

Decision: Total condemnation.

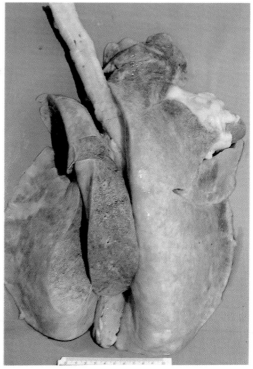

582

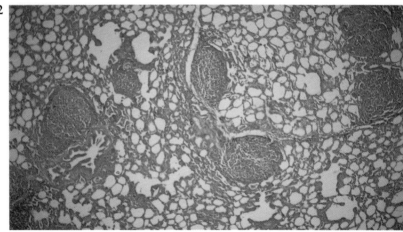

582 Interstitial pneumonia – lung: sheep Progressive interstitial pneumonia where, apart from a moderate thickening of the interalveolar septa, an abnormal proliferation of the lymphoid tissue was taking place, assuming a clear folicular arrangement. H. & E.

583

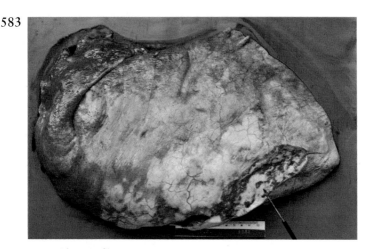

583 Chronic fibrous pneumonia – lung: horse The lungs, which did not collapse after the chest had been opened, had a rubber-like consistency, and whitish areas, whose section showed to be made up of lardaceous shiny tissue.

Decision: Approval with elimination of the lungs.

584 Actinobacillosis – lung: cattle The incision of some firm areas in the lungs revealed the presence of golden-yellow prominent nodules, surrounded by fibrous tissue.

Differential diagnosis: Tuberculosis; Nocardiosis; Metastasis of neoplasia.

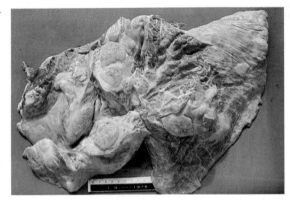

Decision: Total condemnation.
Approval, with elimination of the lungs, can be considered in cases of limited lesions, without lymph node reaction.

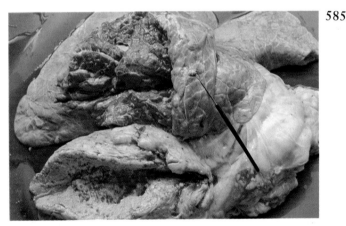

585 Primary complex (tuberculosis) – lung: cattle A small caseous lesion in the diaphragmatic lobe. The mediastinal lymph node showed, on the contrary, extensive caseous lesions with foci of dystrophic calcification.

Differential diagnosis: Actinobacillosis.

Decision: Approval with elimination of the lungs and respective lymph nodes.

586

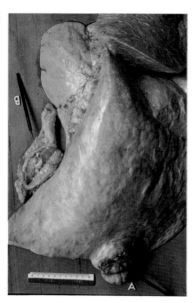

586 Primary complex (tuberculosis) – lung: cattle A small caseous tubercle at the base of the diaphragmatic lobe. The mediastinal lymph node showed calcified caseous lesions. G: mediastinal lymph node.

Differential diagnosis: Actinobacillosis; Non-specific abscess.

Decision: Approval with elimination of the lungs, heart and respective lymph nodes.

587

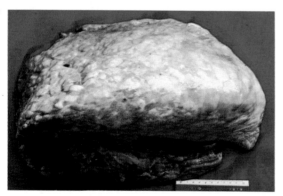

587 Acute miliary tuberculosis – lung: cattle The lungs did not collapse after the opening of the thoracic cavity, due to an emphysema affecting some lobules and interstitial tissue. The aspect of the organ was heterogeneous with lighter emphysema areas and other resembling muscle. Here and there small yellow tubercles could be seen, particularly in the interstitial tissue.

Differential diagnosis: Vesicular emphysema; Metastasis of neoplasia; Actinobacillosis.

Decision: Total condemnation.

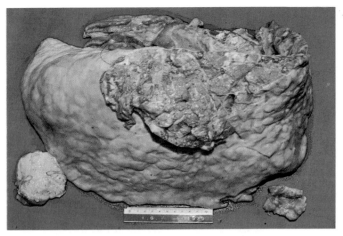

588   Acute miliary tuberculosis – lung: cattle   Section of the lung presented in 587 showing a large number of small caseous tubercles.

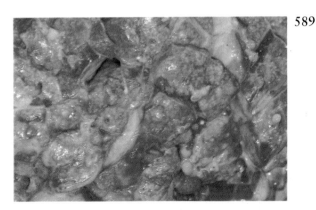

589   Acute miliary tuberculosis – lung: cattle   Greyish tubercles could be seen disseminated in the lung, at the same stage of evolution both in the parenchyma and the interstitial tissue.

Decision: Total condemnation.

590

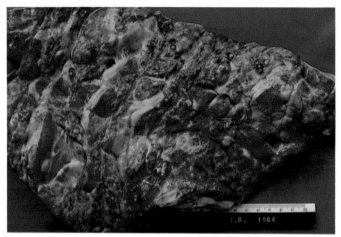

590　Acute miliary tuberculosis – lung: cattle　The incision of
the lungs revealed a multitude of small calcified caseous nodules
in the parenchyma and in the interstitial tissue, which was
distended due to excessive accumulation of air.

Decision: Total condemnation.

591

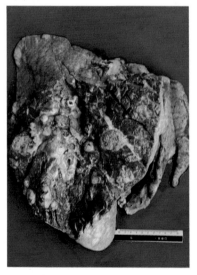

**591　Tuberculosis (acute late
generalization) – breakdown of body
resistance – lung: cattle**　In the
diaphragmatic lobe there are numerous
nodules of various sizes and sharp limits,
surrounded by a fibrous capsule. They
consisted of a shiny tissue, with some
caseous areas and subsequent
calcification. The mediastinal lymph
nodes were hypertrophic due to
extensive calcified caseous lesions
assuming aspects of breakdown of body
resistance.

Differential diagnosis: Actinobacillosis.

Decision: Total condemnation.

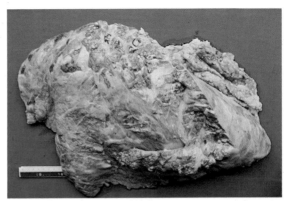

592 Tuberculosis (slow generalization) – lung: cattle Tubercles in different stages of evolution. Side by side with caseous and calcified caseous tubercles were small miliary tubercles and grey tubercles. The lymph nodes of the lung presented lesions all at the same stage of evolution (calcified caseous tubercles).

Differential diagnosis: Actinobacillosis.

Decision: Total condemnation.

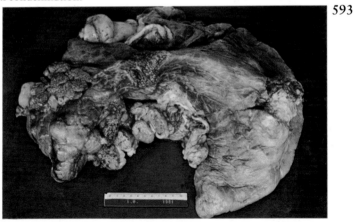

593 Acinar tuberculosis – lung: cattle The cranial part of the diaphragmatic lobe and most of the cranial lobe presented lesions of caseous tuberculosis involving a respiratory bronchioli and the adjacent alveoli. The lesions had in consequence the typical clover-like shape. The lymph nodes presented lesions at the same stage of evolution: breakdown of body resistance.

Decision: Total condemnation.

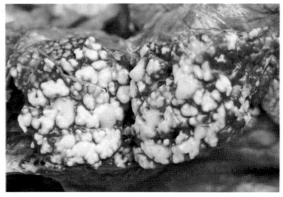

594   Acinar tuberculosis – lung: cattle
Macrophotograph of an area of the lung in 593 showing
the typical clover-like lesions.

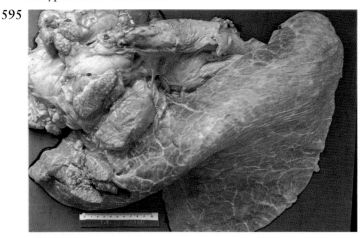

595   Caseous calcified tuberculosis – lung: cattle   A caseous
calcified lesion was identified in the lung. The mediastinal and
bronchial lymph nodes were hypertrophic and showed lesions at
the same stage of evolution. Simultaneously identical lesions were
found in the intestine and in the mesenteric lymph nodes.

Differential diagnosis: Actinobacillosis.

Decision: Total condemnation.
Note: It is possible that the lesions of the intestine and mesenteric
lymph nodes were a consequence of the deglutition of infected
material coming from the lungs.

596 Cavern (chronic tuberculosis) – lung: cattle   In the dorsal margin of the diaphragmatic lobe there is a discrete swelling. Incision showed it was a bronchiectasic cavern, containing mucocaseous matter. The walls of the cavern were congested and smooth with some small tubercles.

Differential diagnosis: Non-tuberculous bronchiectasia.

Decision: Total condemnation.

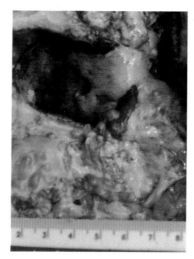

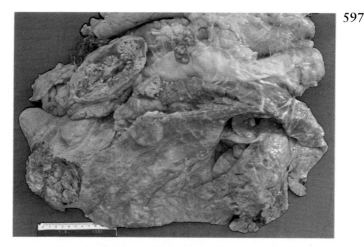

597 Tuberculosis (acute late generalization) – breakdown forms – lung: cattle   The parenchyma showed some calcified caseous lesions surrounded by small tubercles, isolated or in small groups. The lymph nodes presented old calcified lesions together with well-defined small tubercles corresponding to the lesions found in the lungs.

Decision: Total condemnation.

598

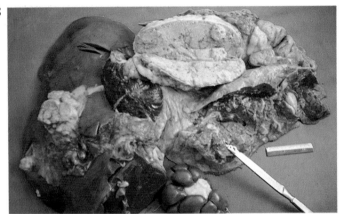

598 Tuberculosis (acute late generalization) – breakdown forms – viscera: cattle   The lung showed discrete lesions in contrast with the highly hypertrophic mediastinal lymph nodes, which were practically destroyed due to extensive lesions of caseous tuberculosis. The kidney and liver were equally affected with calcified caseous lesions of various sizes. The lymph nodes show breakdown lesions.

Decision: Total condemnation.

599

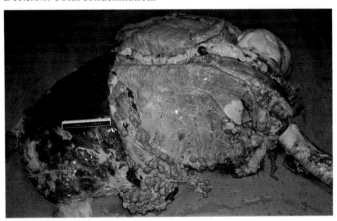

599 Pearl disease (tuberculosis) – viscera: cattle   Productive tuberculous lesions, typically known as 'pearl disease', affecting the visceral pleura, the abdominal surface of the diaphragm and the liver capsule.

Decision: Total condemnation.

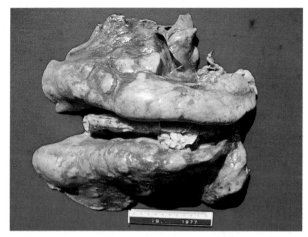

600 Parasitic pneumonia (dictyocaulosis) – lung: sheep The lungs showed a modified profile due to several lighter areas, which were slightly prominent. These were emphysematous areas due to a severe *Dictyocaulus filaria* infection. The parasites filled the bronchial lumen preventing the air from leaving the alveoli.

Differential diagnosis: Adenomatosis.

Decision: Approval with elimination of the lungs.

01 Parasitic pneumonia (dictyocaulosis) lung: sheep A section of the lungs in 600 owing the presence of adult forms of *ictyocaulus filaria* in the large bronchi.

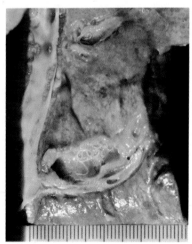

602

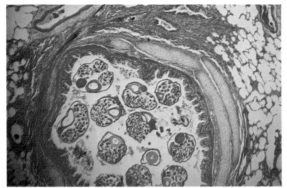

**602 Parasitic bronchopneumonia (dictyocaulus) –
lung: sheep** Several sections of adult parasites in a
large bronchus, the females showing in the uterus large
numbers of embryonated eggs in various stages of
evolution. H. & E.

603

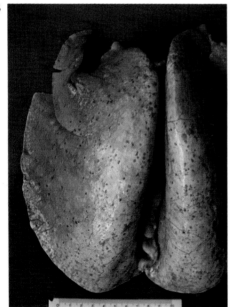

**603 Parasitic pneumonia
(cystocaulosis) – lung: sheep**
These lungs, which did not
collapse when the chest was
opened, were affected by a severe
Cystocaulus ocreatus infection.
The parasites were responsible for
multiple nodules of various
colours, which resemble birdshot
and were easily noticeable under
the pleura.

Differential diagnosis:
Dictyocaulosis; *Muellerius*
infection.

Decision: Approval with
elimination of the lungs.

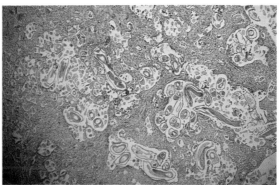

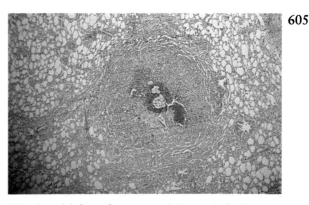

**604   Parasitic bronchopneumonia (cystocaulosis) –
lung: sheep**   This section of the lungs shows the action
of numerous parasites in the bronchi and the alveoli.
Embryonated eggs can also be seen close to the adults or
isolated in small groups in the alveoli. The inflammatory
reaction of the interalveolar septa led to the decrease
of the alveolar capacity. H. & E.

**605   Parasitic bronchopneumonia (cystocaulosis) –
lung: sheep**   Typical nodule of the invasive period with
mixed exudative reactions (around the remains of a
larva) and cellular reactions of the lymphohystiocytic
type. H. & E.

606

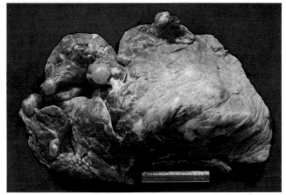

606 Hydatidosis – lung: cattle Various cysts of several sizes at the surface of the lung, containing a colourless fluid. Sectioning revealed membrane structures typical of hydatid cysts.

Decision: Approval with elimination of the lung.

607

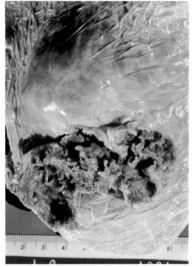

607 Calcified parasitic lesions – lung: cattle The incision of a prominent swelling of the lung revealed necrotic matter, partially calcified, most probably (parasitic nature.

Differential diagnosis: Tuberculosis; Calcinosis pulmonalis; Osteoma.

Decision: Approval with elimination of th affected tissues.

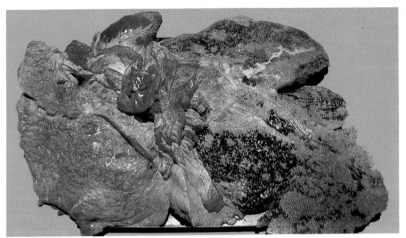

608 Disseminated calcified parasitic nodules – viscera: horse Multiple nodules of milky white colour and hard consistency, deeply modified the appearance of the liver and lungs, which became especially difficult to cut. These changes were due to calcification following a heavy strongyle infection.

Differential diagnosis: Miliary tuberculosis; Neoplasia.

Decision: Approval with elimination of the affected viscera.

609 Adenomatosis – lung: sheep In both cranial lobes and in the dorsal cranial part of the right diaphragmatic lobe there is a solid white tissue with shiny cut surface. This change is commonly named 'white pneumonia'. The tumoral nature is inferred from the frequency of the metastases which develop in the bronchial and mediastinal lymph nodes.

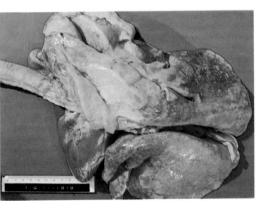

Differential diagnosis: Emphysema in cases of dictyocaulosis.

Decision: Total condemnation.

Some authors support the idea of a viral aetiology. The decision of 'total condemnation' is frequently replaced by less drastic judgements by other authors.

610

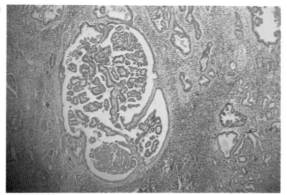

610 Adenomatosis – lung: sheep The metaplasia and
the uncontrolled and invasive proliferation of the
epithelium from the alveoli and terminal bronchioles,
which lead to the functional incapacity of the lungs.
H. & E.

611

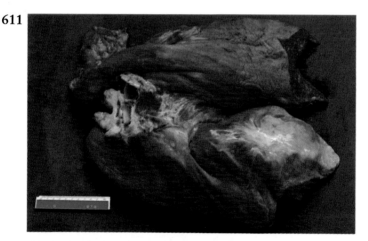

611 Bronchial carcinoma – lung: horse In the posterior
surface of the left diaphragmatic lobe there is a whitish and firm
tumefaction, involving the retraction of the neighbouring tissues
which had a star-like shape typical of malignant neoplasias.

Differential diagnosis: Chronic interstitial pneumonia.

Decision: Total condemnation.

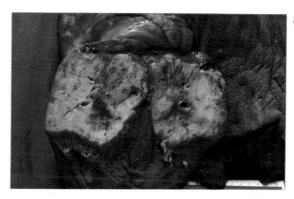

612 Bronchial carcinoma – lung: horse Magnification of the cut surface of the tumour in **611**.

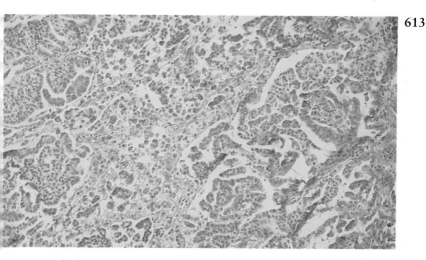

613 Bronchial carcinoma – lung: horse An area of the lung severely invaded by a carcinoma growing from the bronchi. H. & E.

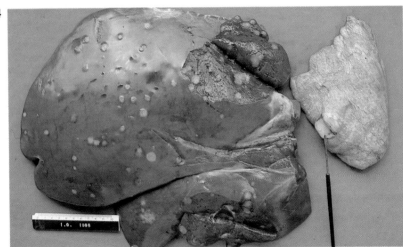

614 Bronchial epidermoid carcinoma – lung and liver: horse Post-mortem, small creamy nodules were seen in the lung. Their incision showed a homogeneous surface area. The liver was seeded with metastatic nodules, clearly seen under the capsule.

Differential diagnosis: Focal necrotic hepatitis; Necrobacillosis; Non-specific granulomas.

Decision: Total condemnation.

615

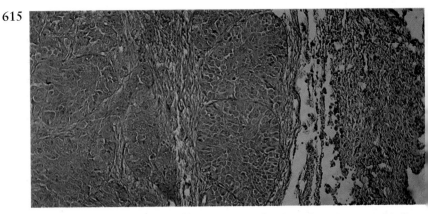

615 Epidermoid carcinoma – lungs: horse The normal respiratory epithelium was replaced by a malpighian epithelium which led to deep changes of the alveolar structures by compression, and to extensive necrotic areas. H. & E.

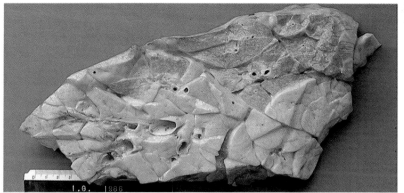

616 Interstitial pneumonia – fragment of lung: cattle A large number of
lobules of the diaphragmatic lobe were affected by interstitial pneumonia, which
gave them a light-colour. Histological examination showed the initial
development of an atypical growth of the bronchial epithelium, sometimes
assuming the appearance of an epidermoid carcinoma.

Decision: Total condemnation.

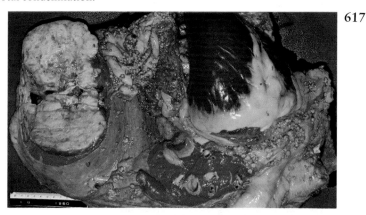

617 Alveolar carcinoma – lung: horse A white and shiny tumour was well
inserted in the lung of a horse. Metastatic dissemination occurred in the serosas
of the thoracic cavity in the heart auricles and in the fat around the heart,
assuming an aspect similar to the serosal pearl disease (tuberculosis).

Differential diagnosis: Pearl disease (tuberculosis); Actinobacillosis; Non-specific
granulomas; Mesothelioma; Chronic interstitial pneumonia.

Decision: Total condemnation.

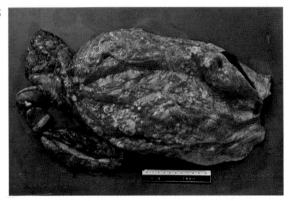

618   Alveolar carcinoma – lung: horse   The palpation of the lungs revealed small firm nodules. They were made up of a whitish-yellow tissue and well disseminated in the parenchyma. The mediastinal lymph nodes were enlarged and bosselated due to large numbers of metastases.

Differential diagnosis: Tuberculosis; Actinobacillosis.

Decision: Total condemnation.

619

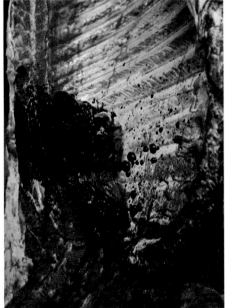

619   Melanotic carcinoma – lung and pleura: horse   Developed from the lung and adherent to the parietal pleura was a black shiny and ill-defined mass, together with small identical neoplasias regularly round or elliptical, which corresponded to metastasis of the neoplasia.

Decision: Total condemnation.

620 Fibroadenocarcinoma – lung: horse The left lung was enlarged and firm and did not collapse after the opening of the chest. The visceral pleura was thickened. The incision showed a lardaceous and haemorrhagic tissue which totally replaced the normal tissue.

Decision: Total condemnation.

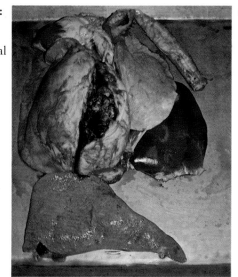

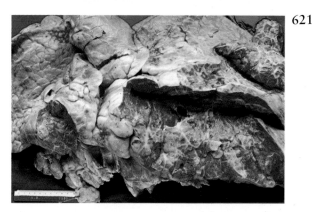

621 Adenocarcinoma – lung: cattle Palpation of the lung revealed vesicular emphysema, and small, firm lumps. The incision showed that some lobules had been replaced by a hard-to-cut yellow-grey tissue. The lymph nodes were equally hardened and their interior characteristics were identical to the tumoral lesions identified in the lung.

Differential diagnosis: Tuberculosis; Actinobacillosis.

Decision: Total condemnation.

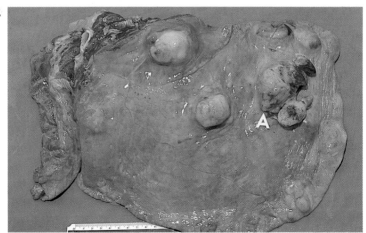

622 Renal adenocarcinoma, metastasis – lung: horse On the surface of the diaphragmatic lobe several greyish/white prominent nodules could be seen, a few centimetres in diameter. The incision made in one of the nodules (A) showed a shiny neoplastic tissue, firm and lardaceous.

Differential diagnosis: Actinobacillosis; Nodular tuberculosis; Pleuropneumonia sequestra.

Decision: Total condemnation.

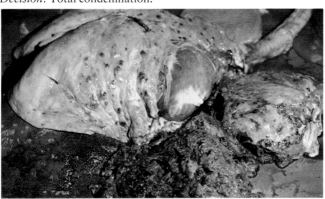

623 Reticulosarcoma – lung: horse From the cranial lobe of the right lung a globular encapsulated neoplasia originated, whose section showed a spongy structure and variegated colour, due to the presence of several haemorrhages. The remaining pulmonary tissue presented small dark-red patches, clearly defined, which resulted from metastatic dissemination of the original tumour.

Decision: Total condemnation.

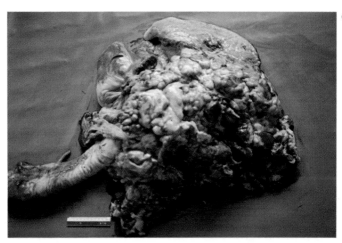

624   Undifferentiated cell sarcoma – lung: cattle   The cranial areas of both lungs were completely destroyed and replaced by a lardaceous, friable and highly vascularized tissue with necrotic foci and haemorrhages. The visceral pleura of the same area was totally destroyed and the tumour had invaded extensive areas of the parietal pleura.

Decision: Total condemnation.

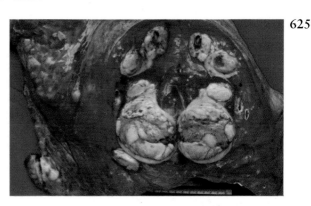

625

625   Undifferentiated cell sarcoma, metastasis – lung: horse   The incision of this enlarged lung of irregular profile, showed numerous tumours, lardaceous and with a necrotic centre. They corresponded to metastasis of an undifferentiated cell sarcoma of the spleen.

Decision: Total condemnation.

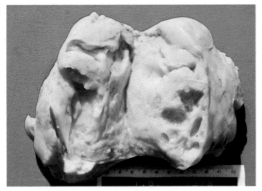

626 Spindle cell sarcoma – mediastinum: sheep
A well-encapsulated neoplasia adhering to the
mediastinum through a connective tissue pedicle.
It is firm and yellow and its section revealed small
empty cavities without a limiting wall.

Differential diagnosis: Lipoma.

Decision: Total condemnation.

627

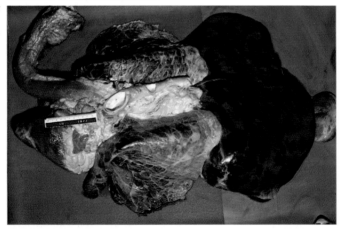

627 Diffuse melanosis – viscera: cattle The lesions, which
resulted from an abnormal genesis of melanotic pigment, were
extremely expressive in the liver, heart and lungs of a calf. The
lungs that were particularly involved were deep black.

Decision: Total condemnation.

628   Melanosis – pleura: cattle The parietal sheath was infiltrated by a black shiny pigment with the characteristics of melanin. Localization in a simple case of melanosis.

Decision: Approval with elimination of the affected pleura.

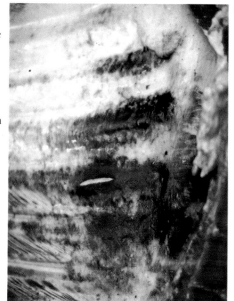

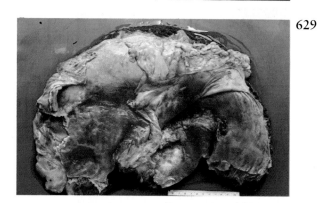

629   Inflammatory reaction – pleura: cattle   An acute inflammatory reaction affected the pleura over the diaphragm. Congestion, haemorrhage and severe serofibrinous exudation were noticed. In some areas proliferative changes were already taking place shown by the fine granular appearance of the serosal surface.

Decision: Approval with elimination of the affected tissues.

337

630

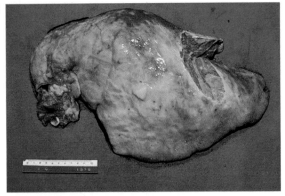

630   Emphysema and pachypleuritis – pleura and lung:
cattle   This lung was distended due to generalized
emphysema. The pleura was affected by a chronic
inflammatory process with clear fibrous thickening,
although small areas of acute pleuritis could be noticed,
with prevalence of congestive reactions.

Decision: Approval with elimination of the lungs.

631

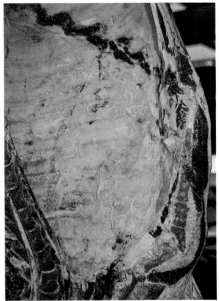

631   Fibrinous pleuritis – pleura:
cattle   The parietal pleura is almos
totally affected by an exudative
inflammatory reaction with build-u
of fibrin. It was only in the dorsal
caudal part that a reduced area of th
pleura remained normal.

Decision: Total condemnation or,
alternatively, approval after heat
treatment, subject to the laboratory
examination results and the animal'
general condition.

632 Fibrinous pleuritis lung: cattle In the left cardiac lobe the pleura was affected by an exudative inflammatory reaction, with deposition of fibrin, which took on a honeycomb-like appearance. In the diaphragmatic lobe the process was older with clear organizational aspects.

The regional lymph nodes were enlarged and moist.

Decision: Total condemnation.

633 Fibrinous purulent pleuroperitonitis – pleura and peritoneum: cattle A large amount of yellow fibrinous and purulent exudate was adherent to the parietal pleura. The peritoneum showed more advanced lesions in some areas, with organizational signs. The reactive sternal lymph nodes could be clearly seen.

Decision: Total condemnation.

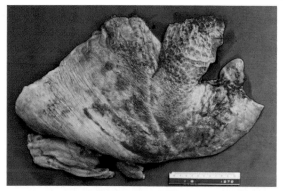

632

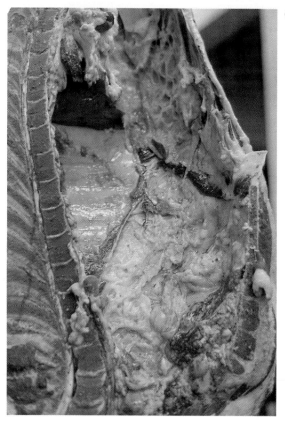

633

339

634

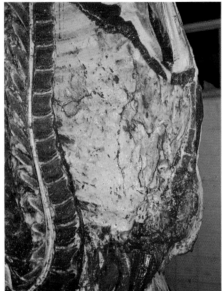

634 Suppurative pleuritis – pleu cattle The pleura was affected by chronic purulent inflammatory reaction and marked fibrosis, lead to multiple symphysis between the pleural layers. The regional lymph nodes were clearly hypertrophic.

Decision: Total condemnation.

635

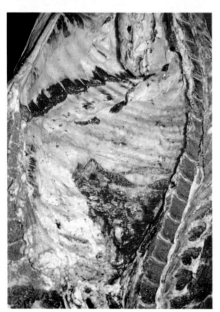

635 Chronic pleuritis – pleura: cattle A chronic inflammatory reaction of the pleura. Extensive symphysis of connective tissue were formed between the pleural layers in such a way that part of the lung was dilacerated when the organ was removed, remaining adherent to the costal wall.

Decision: Approval with elimination of the affected tissues.

636 Pearl disease, tuberculosis – pleura: cattle Most of the parietal pleura, particularly in the sternal region, was invaded by multiple nodules, some the size of a pea and others more voluminous, pinkish and assuming in some areas a cauliflower-like appearance.

Differential diagnosis: actinobacillosis; Metastasis of neoplasia.

Decision: Total condemnation.

637 Cysticercosis (*Cysticercus tenuicollis*) – pleura: sheep Several pediculated vesicles adhere to the visceral pleura of a sheep. They had a clear content and transparent wall, through which a white granule, corresponding to an invaginated scolex, could be seen. The heart's hydropic fat reveals the animal's poor condition.

Differential diagnosis: Mesothelioma (with cystic degeneration).

Decision: Total condemnation, due to the heavy parasitic infection and the general poor condition.

Note: The carcases of animals in good condition are approved, with elimination of the affected parts or organs.

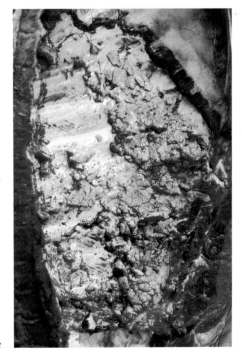

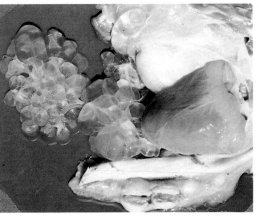

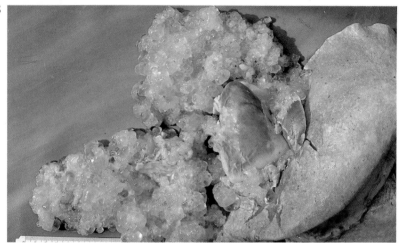

638 Mesothelioma with cystic degeneration – pleura: sheep A mesothelioma developed from the pleura, with a cystic appearance. The cysts show a clear fluid content, similar to water.

Differential diagnosis: Infestation with *Cysticercus tenuicollis*.

Decision: Total condemnation.

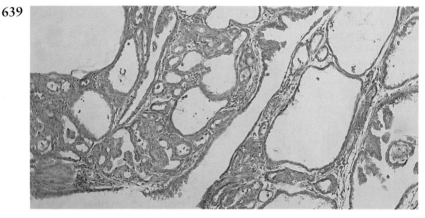

639 Mesothelioma with cystic degeneration – pleura: sheep The tumour arose from the pleural serosa, assuming a cystic shape, considered typical of such tumours. H. & E.

8: The urinary system

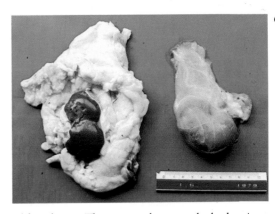

640 Hydropic fat – perirenal fat: sheep   The contrast between the hydropic aspect of the perirenal fat in a cachectic animal (right) and the perirenal fat of a normally fed animal (left).

Differential diagnosis: Perirenal oedema.

Decision: Total condemnation in case of hydrocachexia.

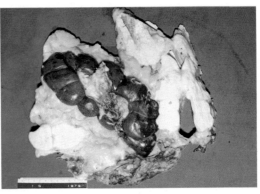

641 Necrosis of the perirenal fat: cattle   The white necrotic areas were hard to cut and had a dry cut surface. This is a focal regressive change, which in this case affected the perirenal fat.

Decision: Approval, with elimination of the affected perirenal fat.

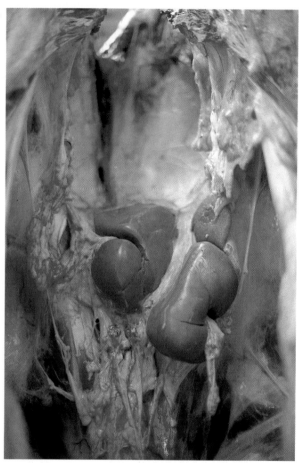

642 Dystopia – kidney: horse The carcase did not present particular changes except for the abnormal localization of the kidneys which were in the pelvis.

Decision: Approval.

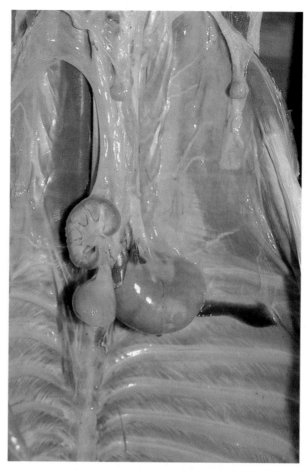

643 Unilateral renal atrophy – kidney: sheep The kidneys showed abnormal volume due to atrophy of the cortex, which was only a few millimetres thick, in contrast to the heterolateral organ which showed a compensatory hypertrophy.

Decision: Approval of carcase and offal with exclusion of the kidneys.

644

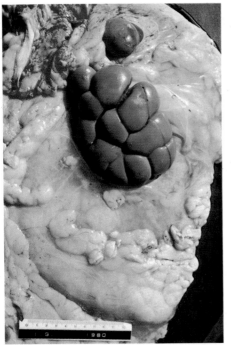

644 Perirenal oedema – kidney: cattle This well-covered kidney was separated from the surrounding fat by a transparent fluid, that rapid tests revealed to be rich in proteins. The aetiology was unknown.

Decision: Approval, if no other lesions are present, with elimination of the kidney. Perirenal oedema is frequent in the course of nephrosis whose aetiology is thought to be related to endogenous or exogenous toxins. Intoxication by mercury, arsenic, oxalates, overdoses of sulphamides and above all feeding with the plant *Amaranthus retroflexus* may cause nephrosis, which leads to severe perirenal oedema in cattle or swine.

645

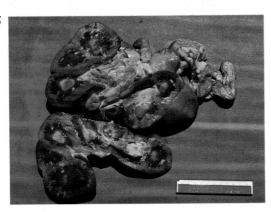

645 Malformation – kidney: cattle This kidney's deformity approached the shape of th' horseshoe kidney. The existence of the other kidney proved that it was not a congenital disturbance. Infarct-like lesions were noticed in the cut surface.

Decision: Approval with elimination of the kidney.

346

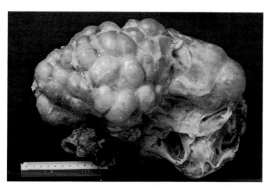

646 Hydronephrosis – kidney: cattle Numerous large cysts were seen at the surface of the kidney, containing a clear fluid. This change was due to mechanical obstruction of the ureter, with consequent retention of urine. Only one kidney was affected.

Differential diagnosis: Pyelonephritis; Polycystic kidney (congenital); Renal cysts.

Decision: Approval with elimination of the affected kidney.

647

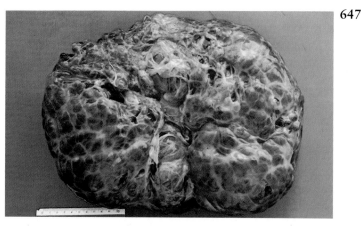

647 Hydronephrosis – kidney: sheep The surface of the kidney was bosselated due to multiple cysts which transformed the kidney into a thin-walled sac containing a yellowish fluid. This disturbance is frequently unilateral.

Differential diagnosis: Polycystic kidney.

Decision: Approval with elimination of the kidney.

648

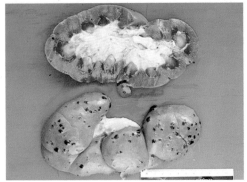

648   Cysts – kidney: cattle   Small cysts were disseminated on the kidney surface, slightly raised under the capsule, containing a dark-brown liquid.

Decision: Approval with elimination of the kidney.

649

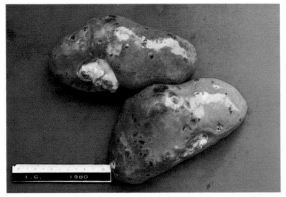

649   Cysts – kidney: swine   Cysts of various sizes could be seen under the capsule.

Decision: Approval with elimination of the kidney.

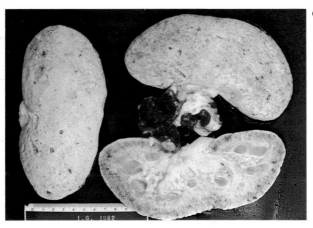

650 Polycystic kidney: swine This yellow-straw coloured kidney showed the cortex filled by large numbers of small cavities which gave it a typical spongy appearance.

Decision: Approval with elimination of the kidneys.
A high percentage of animals from the same lot presented similar kidney lesions, which suggests a hereditary problem.

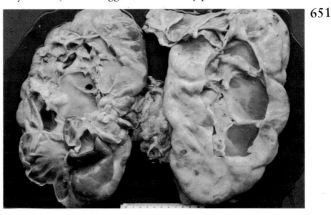

651 Polycystic kidney: swine Advanced case of polycystic kidney. In most of the organ the functional tissue was reduced to a fibrous capsule and the remaining parenchyma was no more than 1 mm thick.

Decision: Total condemnation due to the smell of urine in the meat.

652

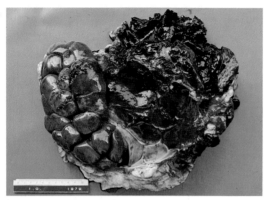

652   Fracture – kidney: cattle   The renal
parenchyma presented various fractures of traumatic
origin, which explains the large perirenal
haematoma.

Decision: Approval with elimination of the affected
kidney.

653

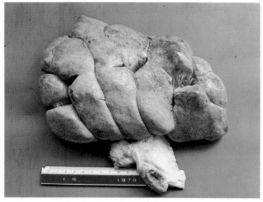

653   Fat necrosis – kidney: cattle   The kidneys were enlarged, yellow and with
soft consistency. After removal of the capsule the parenchyma felt greasy.

Differential diagnosis: Amyloidosis.

Decision: Approval, if no other lesions are present and if there is no general effect
on the carcase, with elimination of the kidneys.

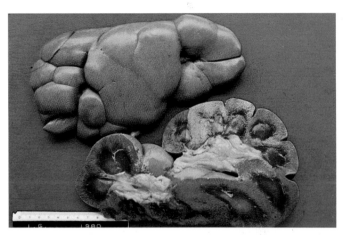

654 Lipoid nephrosis – kidney: cattle The surface of the kidney was abnormally brown. The incision showed that the lesions were confined to the cortex, the colour of the medulla being normal. This change was due to a severe accumulation of fat in cells of the convoluted tubules.

Differential diagnosis: Amyloidosis.

Decision: Approval with elimination of the kidneys.

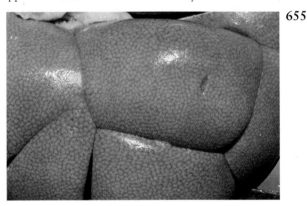

655 Lipoid nephrosis – kidney: cattle This macrophotograph of **655** shows a fine reticular pattern due to the fat infiltration of the cells of the convoluted ducts, which gives them a light yellow colour contrasting with the red-brown interstitial tissue.

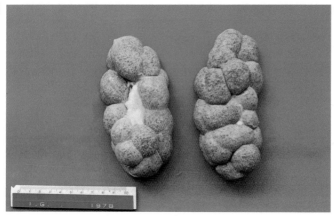

656 Urate deposits – kidney: cattle   The greyish colour of the kidneys was due to the accumulation of urates in the tubules of the cortex. The surface of the organ looked granular with a fine reticular pattern.

Decision: Approval with elimination of the kidneys.

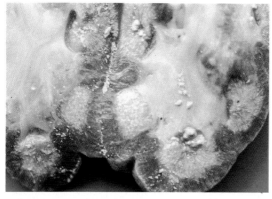

657 Urate deposits – kidney: cattle   This macrophotograph of **656** shows that some tubules of the cortex contain small nodular structures, particularly just under the capsule. In the medulla the accumulation of urates was more severe, assuming aspects of lithiasis.

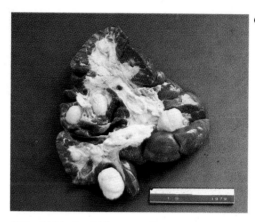

658   Lithiasis – kidney: cattle   Inserted in the calyces, four large yellow calculi could be seen, compressing the parenchyma.

Decision: Approval with elimination of the kidney.

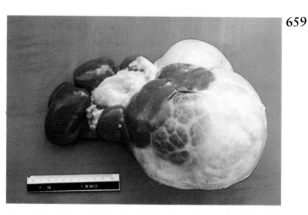

659   Renal cyst following lithiasis – kidney: cattle
Two different, but possibly related changes were noted at the surface of this kidney: two large cysts and small nodules in the cortex. These corresponded to calculi which might have been there at the formation of the cysts, due to obstruction of renal ducts.

Decision: Approval with elimination of the kidney.

660

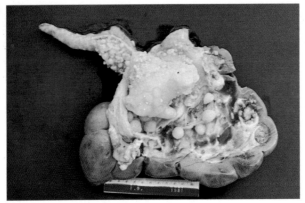

660   Lithiasis – kidney: cattle   A large polylobated calculus in the pelvis extended into the ureter, causing its occlusion. Several spherical calculi of various dimensions were located in the calyces area. The medulla on the right side is atrophic due to the presence of the calculi.

Decision: Approval with elimination of the kidney.

661

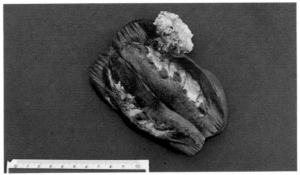

661   Lithiasis – kidney: swine   A single calculus was formed in the pelvis. Its growth led to the fracture of the kidney and capsule, giving the calculus a bush-like appearance.

Decision: Approval with elimination of the kidney.

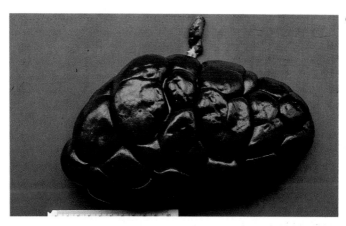

662 Haemosiderosis – kidney: cattle This slightly swollen kidney was dark-brown due to the accumulation of haemosiderin, an iron pigment derived from the haemoglobin, which infiltrates the cells of the convoluted tubules. This may occur during infectious or parasitic diseases involving haemolysis, intoxication and metabolic disturbances. The renal lymph node was equally infiltrated by haemosiderin.

Differential diagnosis: Haemocromatosis; Porphyria; Infiltration by lipofuscin.

Decision: Approval with elimination of the kidneys.

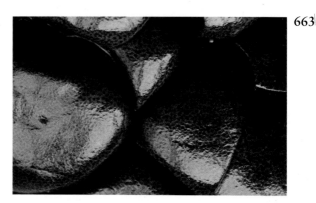

663 Haemosiderosis – kidney: cattle This macrophotograph of **662** shows a characteristic honeycomb-like pattern, with small dark-brown patches, surrounded by a brownish-yellow tissue.

664

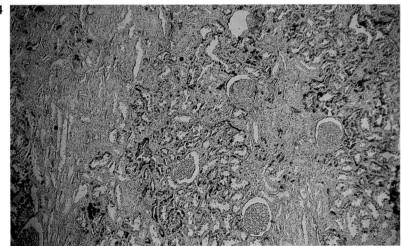

664 Haemosiderosis – kidney: cattle Most cortical tubules presented the cells filled with blood-derived pigment (haemosiderin). The pigment, stained with Prussian blue, covers and hides the nuclei of the tubular cells. Prussian blue.

665

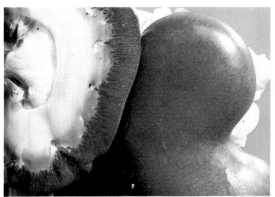

665 Haemosiderosis – kidney: sheep This macrophotograph of a kidney's cut surface shows three areas of distinct colours: a cortex with dark-brown strands running up to the medulla, which are typical of haemosiderosis; a salmon-pink outer medulla; and a plain yellow inner medulla.

Decision: Approval with elimination of the kidneys.

666 Methaemoglobinaemia kidney: cattle The kidney was deeply black due to the infiltration of the tubular cells by a blood-derived pigment, which contains iron in the ferric form.

Differential diagnosis: Lipofuscinosis; Haemosiderosis; Cholaemic nephrosis.

Decision: Approval, if no other lesions are present, with elimination of the kidneys.

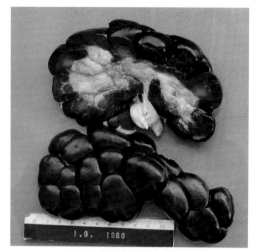

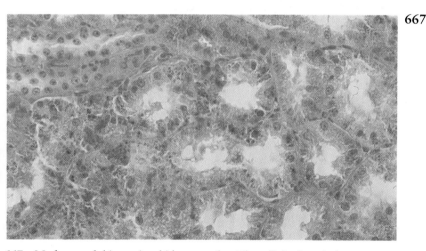

667 Methaemoglobinaemia – kidney: cattle The cells in the tubules, apart from degenerative changes, also show large amounts of brown pigment, which was probably methaemoglobin. H. & E.

668

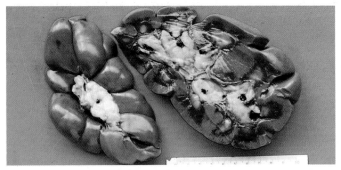

668 Melanosis – kidney: cattle In the hilum of the kidney, a small black nodule was noticed as well as dark patches on the surface of the organ. The section of the kidney showed that the fat in the pelvis was infiltrated with melanin, sometimes in a cord-like fashion or in nodules. Identical lesions were found in the lungs, pleura, heart, blood vessels and lymph nodes.

Decision: Total condemnation considering the generalization. Melanin may be bleached by oxidizing agents such as hydrogen peroxide, potassium permanganate, etc., which can be used for diagnostic purposes.

669

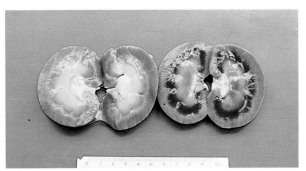

669 Cholaemic nephrosis – kidney: sheep The organ on the left, contrasts with the normal one on the right. It shows a greenish-yellow colour, particularly in the medulla and pelvis due to the infiltration of biliary pigments in a case of jaundice. The cortex, equally infiltrated, was affected by cholaemic nephrosis.

Differential diagnosis: Amyloidosis; Lipoid nephrosis.

Decision: Total condemnation (jaundice).

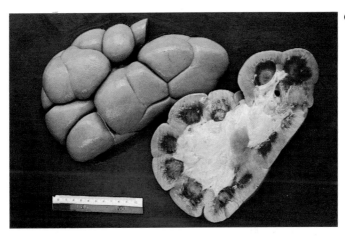

670 Amyloidosis – kidney: cattle The kidney, which was slightly hypertrophic and had an easily removable capsule, was pale with a shiny cortex, suggesting amyloidosis. In cases such as this the deposition of a yellow ochre pigment in the convoluted tubules occurs frequently.

Differential diagnosis: Lipoid nephrosis; Secondary amyloidosis.

Decision: Total condemnation.

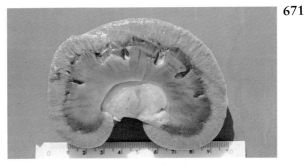

671 Amyloidosis – kidney: sheep This slightly swollen kidney had a golden-yellow cortex due to the deposition of amyloid, particularly in the glomerulus and in the adventitia of the small cortical blood vessels.

Differential diagnosis: Infiltration of fat; Cholaemic nephrosis; Secondary amyloidosis.

Decision: Total condemnation.

672

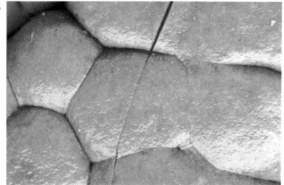

672 Amyloidosis – kidney: cattle This kidney shows
numerous yellow ochre patches at the surface of the
kidney. They were thought to be due to a water soluble
pigment, because it was not possible to identify them in
the tubules in histological sections stained with
haematoxylin and eosin.
A macroscopic test – Lugol's iodine – can be used in
inspection to demonstrate the presence of amyloid.

673

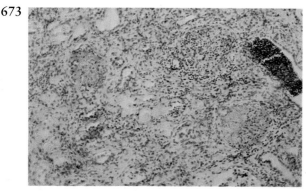

673 Amyloidosis – kidney: cattle The glomerular
capillaries almost filled the Bowman's space due to the
deposition of amyloid in their basement membrane.
Similar deposits could be seen around small interstitial
vessels. Congo red.

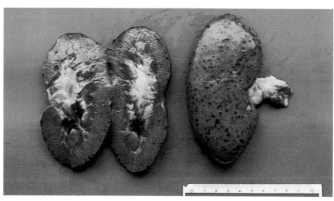

674 Haemorrhages (African swine fever) – kidney: swine The kidney showed haemorrhages in the cortex, particularly just under the capsule. They were small haemorrhages slightly larger than the petechiae typical of hog cholera. More extensive haemorrhages were seen in the pelvis.

Virology: African swine fever virus.

Differential diagnosis: Hog cholera; Erysipelas.

Decision: Total condemnation.

675

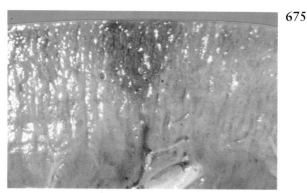

675 Ischaemic infarct – kidney: swine The incision of the kidney showed a small dark triangle, corresponding to a recent infarct. The dilated intralobular artery can be seen in the macrophotograph, with blood accumulating upstream the point of obstruction. This is usually caused by an embolus.

Decision: Approval with elimination of the lesion or of the whole kidney.

676

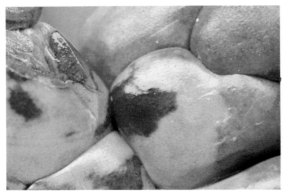

676   Focal necrosis – kidney: cattle   A few red necrotic foci were identified at the surface of the kidney, which penetrated, wedge-like, more or less deeply into the cortex.

Decision: Approval with elimination of the kidney.

677

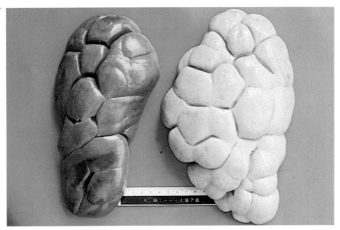

677   Subacute glomerulonephritis (enlarged and pale kidney) – kidney: cattle   The kidney on the right is considerably enlarged and pale. The capsule was easily removed, revealing a fine granular cortex. The normal kidney on the left was obtained from a carcase with approximately the same weight.

Differential diagnosis: Cloudy swelling; Nephrosis.

Decision: Approval with elimination of the kidneys.

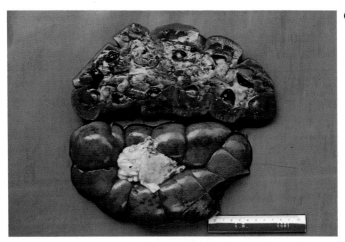

678 Interstitial nephritis – kidney: cattle Congestion and haemorrhages were noticed at the surface of the organ. In the cortex and medulla, which were atrophic, thin pale strands could be seen. More or less extensive haemorrhages in the calyces were compressing the papillae. The pelvis was abnormally large and filled with fat tissue.

Decision: Approval with elimination of the kidneys.

679 Subacute interstitial nephritis – kidney: swine The surface of the kidney was irregular due to small white subcapsular nodules which corresponded to foci of subacute interstitial nephritis. The more or less deep grooves noticed in the cortex were formed as a consequence of cicatricial retraction of older areas of infection.

Decision: Approval with elimination of the kidneys.

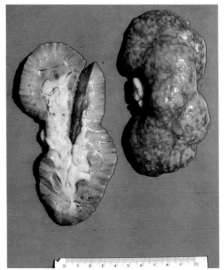

680

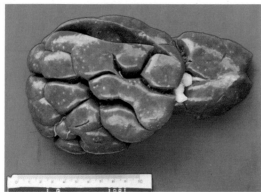

680 Focal interstitial nephritis – kidney: cattle
After removal of the capsule, large numbers of small yellow nodules were seen in the cortex, which corresponded to foci of interstitial nephritis.

Differential diagnosis: Miliary tuberculosis; Lithiasis.

Decision: Approval with elimination of the kidneys.

681

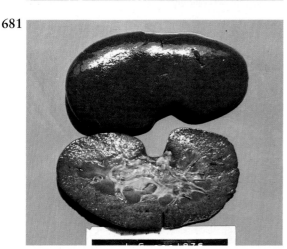

681 Acute glomerulonephritis – kidney: swine This kidney was enlarged and the capsule was easily removed. Small dark dots could be seen in the reddish cortex. The incision showed congestion involving both cortex and medulla. The histopathological examination confirmed the existence of acute glomerulonephritis, with congestion of the glomerular capillaries and haemorrhages in the Bowman's space.

Differential diagnosis: Erysipelas.

Decision: Total condemnation.
Note: Several lymph nodes from the carcase and viscera showed reactive changes (septicaemia).

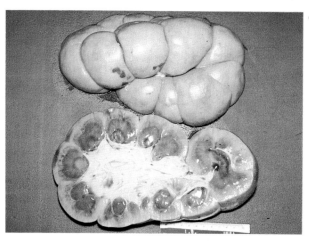

682   Chronic glomerulonephritis – kidney: cattle   This slightly swollen kidney was pale and after removal of the capsule the surface was seen to be finely granular. The incision showed a thinner cortex and the corticomedullar limits not well defined.

Differential diagnosis: Amyloidosis; Lipoid nephrosis.

Decision: Approval with elimination of the kidneys.

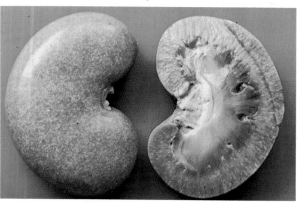

683   Chronic glomerulonephritis – kidney: sheep   The kidney's size was normal but the colour was yellowish-grey. Under the capsule, fine whitish spots covered the cortex, corresponding to sclerosis involving the glomeruli and small areas of surrounding parenchyma.

Decision: Approval with elimination of the kidneys.

684

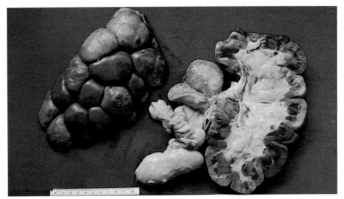

684 Chronic glomerulonephritis and abscesses – kidney: cattle The removal of the capsule uncovered a heterogeneous parenchyma, with aspects of chronic glomerulonephritis in some lobes alternating with normal lobes. The surface of one of the lobes was deformed by microabscesses. The renal and lumbar lymph nodes were also involved.

685

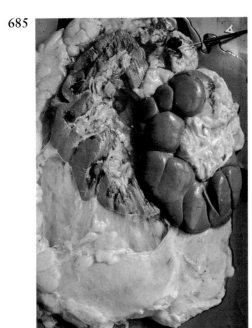

Differential diagnosis: Tuberculosis

Decision: Total condemnation.

685 Subacute glomerulonephritis and perirenal oedema – kidney: cattle The kidney which was affected by subacute glomerulonephritis was surrounded by a considerable amount of a transparent fluid, that easily drained when the tissues were sectioned.

Differential diagnosis: Hydropic perirenal fat in hydrocachexia.

Decision: Approval with elimination of the kidney and surrounding fat (including the adrenal gland).

686 Non-suppurative interstitial nephritis – white spotted kidney: cattle   The cortex presented a series of white nodules whose diameter varied from a few millimetres to 1 cm. These lesions are typical of focal interstitial nephritis occurring in calves, but not common in adult animals. The regional lymph nodes were slightly swollen.

Differential diagnosis: Metastasis of neoplasia; Nodular tuberculosis.

Decision: Approval with elimination of the kidneys.

Note: In this particular case the carcase and viscera were condemned due to antibiotic residues.

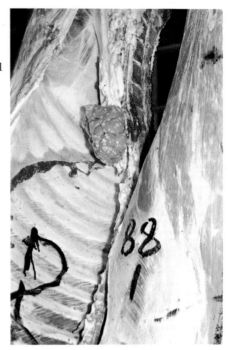

687 Non-suppurative interstitial nephritis – white spotted kidney: cattle   The section of the kidney from **686** shows that the lesions were mainly cortical. They are usually prominent under the capsule and penetrate more or less deeply into the medulla, sometimes up to the papillae.

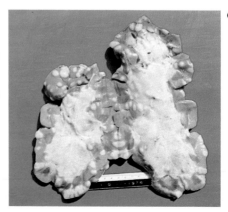

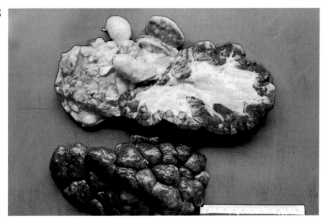

688 Chronic nephritis – kidney: cattle This slightly reduced kidney showed a dark-brown colour interrupted in a few lobes by areas of whitish tissue, visible through the capsule. The sclerosis alternating with normal tissue produced a typical appearance of 'wrinkled' kidney. White strands in the thin cortical tissue can be seen in the cut surface of the organ. The regional lymph nodes were hypertrophic.

Bacteriological examination of the renal lymph nodes: This was negative.

Decision: Approval with elimination of the kidneys.

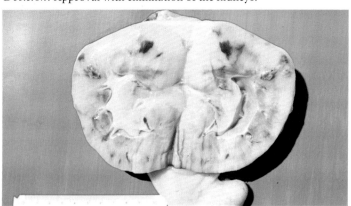

689 Chronic interstitial nephritis – kidney: sheep The whole kidney was extremely pale, particularly the cortex just under the capsule. A small well-defined necrotic foci was identified in the cortex. The renal lymph node was hypertrophic.

Decision: Approval with elimination of both kidneys.

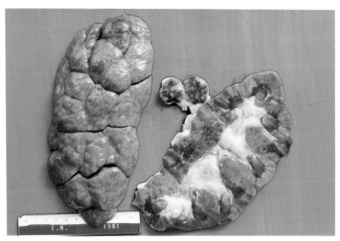

690 Chronic interstitial nephritis – kidney: cattle The surface of the kidney was irregular due to multiple lesions of scar contraction. The cortex was reduced and run by thin whitish strands. The pelvis had a considerable amount of fat tissue.

Decision: Approval with elimination of both kidneys.

691

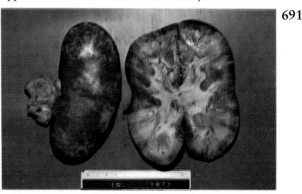

691 Chronic interstitial nephritis – kidney: swine The kidney showed a succession of pale zones and scar retraction areas. In the cut surface, it could be seen that wedge-like pale strands of fibrous tissue ran from the cortex more or less deeply into the medulla.

Decision: Approval with elimination of both kidneys.

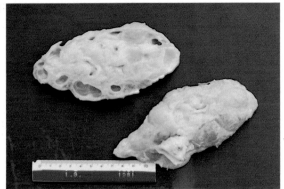

**692 Chronic interstitial nephritis – kidney:
cattle** The organ was extremely pale due to the
replacement of normal by fibrous tissue. The incision
showed a few large cysts due to urinary retention.

Decision: Approval with elimination of both kidneys.

693

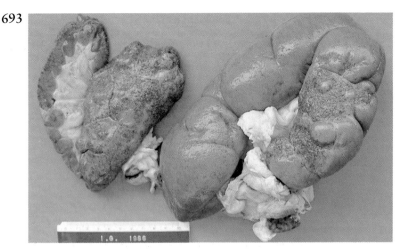

693 Chronic interstitial nephritis – kidney with haemosiderosis: cattle One of
the kidneys was atrophic due to reduction of the parenchyma. The fine granular
surface was dark-brown due to the infiltration of considerable amounts of
haemosiderin. The other kidney was equally affected in small restricted areas.

Decision: Approval with elimination of both kidneys.

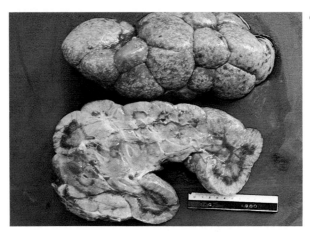

694 Embolic purulent nephritis – kidney: cattle Yellow microabscesses were disseminated throughout the entire pale cortex.
Bacteriological examination of the kidney: This showed *Proteus mirabilis.*

Decision: Total condemnation.

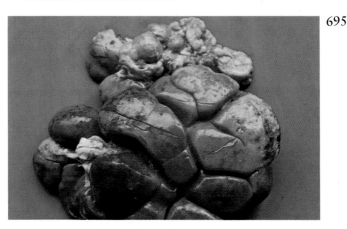

695 Embolic purulent nephritis – kidney: cattle Multiple yellow abscesses of various sizes were noticed at the surface of the kidney, surrounded by a congestive halo. The renal and lumbar lymph nodes were enlarged.

Decision: Total condemnation.

696

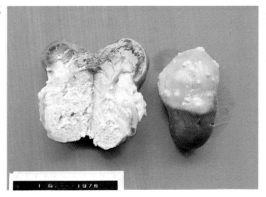

696 Purulent nephritis – kidney: sheep Half of both kidneys was replaced by yellowish-grey purulent matter, odourless and pasty.

Bacteriological examination of the kidneys: This showed *Streptococcus betahaemolyticus.*

Decision: Total condemnation.

697

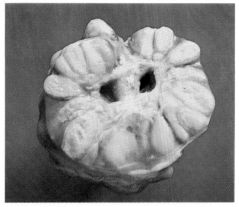

697 Purulent nephritis – kidney: sheep The cross-section of the bosselated kidney uncovered multiple abscesses of fibrous wall, containing a golden-yellow creamy pus.

Decision: Total condemnation.

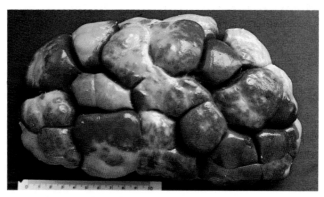

698 **Pyelonephritis – kidney: cattle**   The kidney was hypertrophic and showed under the capsule (removal of which was difficult) whitish-yellow patches of variable diameter, some occupying an entire lobe. Small irregular retractions were noticed at the surface of some lobes corresponding to a retraction of fibrous tissue which replaced a considerable amount of the normal parenchyma.
Decision: Approval with elimination of both kidneys.
Note: Approval was justified due to the non-existence of other lesions in the carcase or remaining viscera.

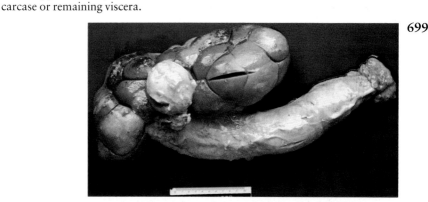

699 **Pyelonephritis and ureteritis – kidney and ureter: cattle**
The ureter was dilated as a consequence of an inflammatory lesion noticeable at the distal end and which caused its obstruction. The kidney showed typical lesions of pyelonephritis (ascending infection) originating in the ureter.

Decision: Approval with elimination of the kidney and ureter.
Note: The lesion was unilateral and no other changes were present in the carcase or remaining viscera.

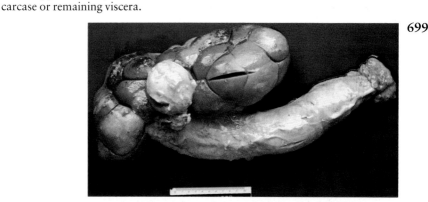

700

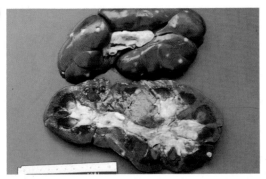

700 Tuberculosis (slow generalization of primary infection) – kidney: cattle   A few caseous nodules, the size of a pea, were noticed in the cortex, less in number and greater in size than the nodules in acute miliary tuberculosis. The renal lymph nodes showed calcified caseous lesions.

Differential diagnosis: Focal interstitial nephritis of the calf; Metastasis of neoplasia.

Decision: Total condemnation.

701

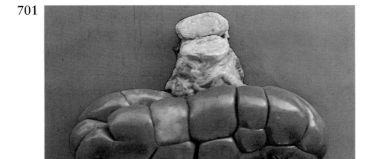

701 Tuberculosis – caseating medullary nephritis (breakdown of body resistance) – kidney: cattle   These lesions are typically a breakdown form of tuberculosis, in which the dominating change is caseation, involving most of a single or several renal lobes, showing up as pale strands limited by congestion and haemorrhages. The cortex of the affected lobes is usually pale, yellow or greyish, thin and frequently depressed. Some authors describe these lesions as the 'chessboard' kidney, due to the alternate pale and dark lobes. The lymph node showed concentric rings of caseation.

Differential diagnosis: Focal interstitial nephritis.

Decision: Total condemnation.

374

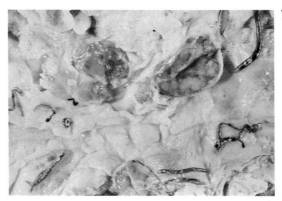

702 Stephanurosis – perirenal fat: swine In the perirenal fat of a swine several *Stephanurus dentatus* nematodes were seen. These parasites live in the kidneys and in the perirenal fat in small galleries and cavities.

Decision: Approval with elimination of the kidneys and perirenal fat.

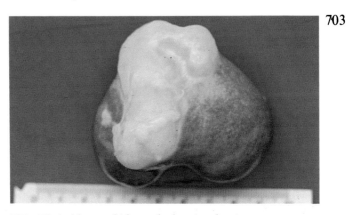

703 Hydatid cyst – kidney: sheep A voluminous cyst, containing a transparent liquid, was observed in the kidney. The identification of membranes and scolices inside the cyst made diagnosis of hydatid cyst possible.

Differential diagnosis: Non-specific renal cyst.

Decision: Approval with elimination of the kidney.

704

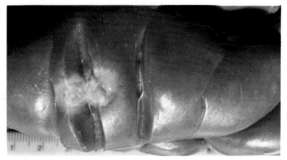

704 Hydatid cyst (purulent involution) – kidney: cattle A small nodule limited by a pale tissue was noticed at the surface of the kidney. The incision showed a granular tissue surrounded by a fibrous capsule.

Differential diagnosis: Nodular tuberculosis.

Decision: Approval with elimination of the kidney.

705

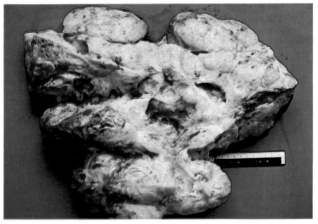

705 Hypernephroma (undifferentiated renal carcinoma) – kidney: sheep This enlarged kidney had a globular shape and its section showed that most of the parenchyma was replaced by a greyish-yellow tissue, solid in some zones and spongy in others, with some haemorrhagic foci. The neoplasia was surrounded by connective tissue arranged as a capsule. These changes were unilateral.

Decision: Total condemnation.

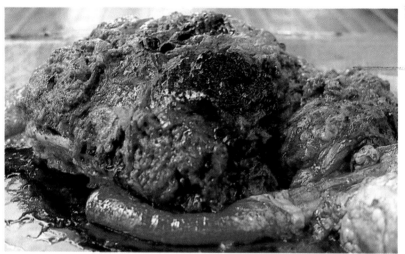

706 Embryonal nephroma – kidney: cattle In the infralumbar region part of a neoplasia weighing 49 kg is shown. It appeared very irregular, poorly defined and highly heterogeneous. Part of the tumour detached during the splitting of the carcase.

Decision: Total condemnation.

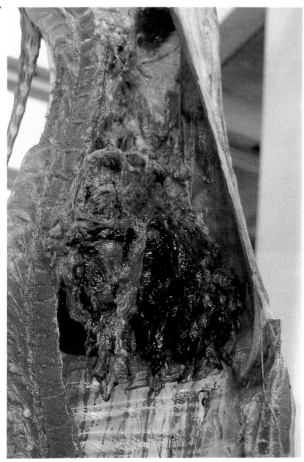

707 **Embryonal nephroma – carcase: cattle** A
complement to the neoplasia in **706**. It showed poorly
defined limits, soft consistency and reddish colour. At the
surface and deeper in the neoplasia several dark-red
haemorrhagic foci could be seen.

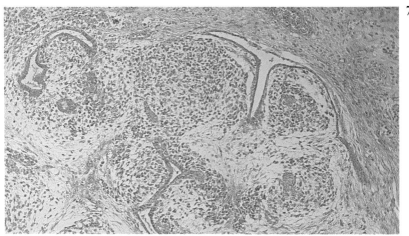

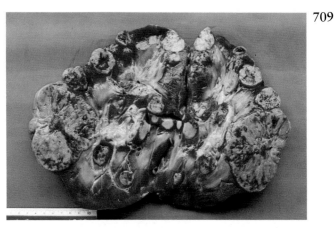

708 **Embryonal nephroma – kidney: cattle**   The neoplasia had structures vaguely similar to glomeruli and renal tubules. H. & E.

709   **Adenocarcinoma – kidney: horse**   A large tumour affecting both cortex and medulla. Smaller well-defined masses with a similar appearance could also be seen, corresponding to metastatic haematogenous generalization. Metastases were furthermore identified in the renal lymph nodes, lungs, heart, spleen and adrenal glands.

Decision: Total condemnation.

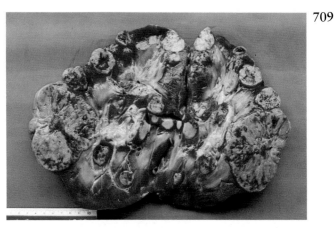

710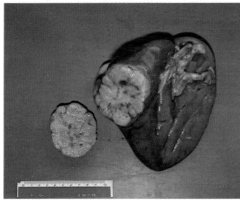

710 Adenocarcinoma – kidney: horse A large pale and prominent nodule was noticed at the surface of the kidney. The incision showed a shiny tissue with some haemorrhagic foci.

Decision: Total condemnation

711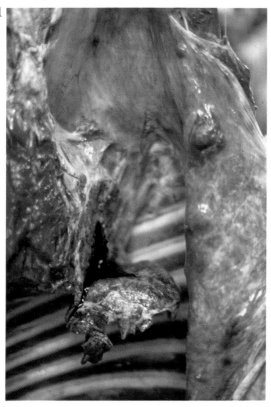

711 Renal carcinoma of papillary pattern – kidney: horse The kidney was partially destroyed as a consequence of the development of a tumour, which deeply modified its profile. The incision showe the renal parenchyma replaced by neoplastic tissue. The parietal peritoneum was congested and invaded by metastasis of the renal neoplasia.

Decision: Total condemnation.

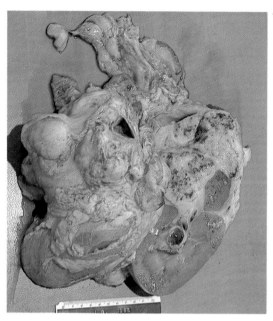

712 Undifferentiated cell adenocarcinoma – kidney: horse At the surface of the kidney rounded masses of variable diameter could be seen, adherent to the involving capsule. The sagittal section of the kidney showed that half the organ was affected.

Differential diagnosis: Interstitial nephritis.

Decision: Total condemnation.

713 Lymphoblastic leukosis – kidney: swine The kidney, yellow due to fatty change, presented several superficial red nodules, of various sizes and regular round profile.

Decision: Total condemnation.
Note: The renal lymph node was enlarged and its cut surface was lardaceous.

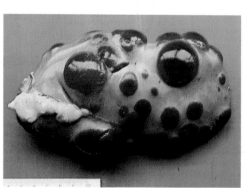

714

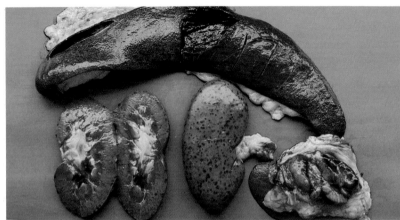

714 African swine fever – viscera: swine The haemorrhages noticeable in the renal cortex and pelvis, the marked congestive haemorrhagic splenomegaly and the discrete haemorrhages in the hepatic lymph nodes are African swine fever lesions, which had not spread, because the course of the disease was interrupted by slaughter and also because of the bleeding.
Decision: Total condemnation.

715

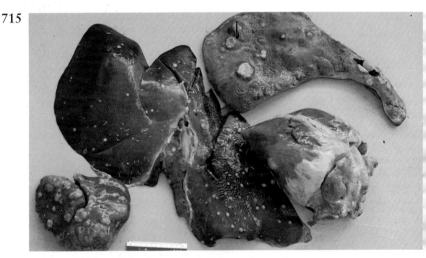

715 Metastatical generalization of neoplasia – viscera: horse The primary tumour, an adenocarcinoma, was located in the kidney. Metastatic spread has affected the lungs and capillary system. The picture shows metastasis in the spleen, heart (rare), liver and in the kidney itself.
Differential diagnosis: Non-specific granulomas.
Decision: Total condemnation.

Urinary bladder

716 Urinary obstruction – urinary bladder: cattle Dilatation of the urinary bladder consecutive to obstruction due to adenomatous proliferation of the bulbourethral glands, which caused occlusion of the urethra.

Differential diagnosis: Retained calculus.

Decision: Approval with elimination of the bladder.

Note: The carcase and viscera did not present any other changes, namely urinary odour.

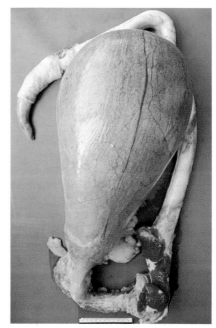

717 Haemorrhagic cystitis – urinary bladder: sheep The urinary bladder, whose walls were thickened, showed a red colour due to external haemorrhagic inflammatory reaction.

Decision: Approval with elimination of the urinary bladder.

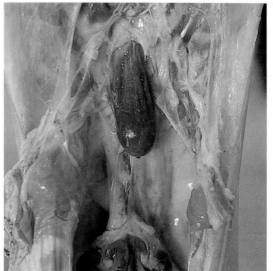

718

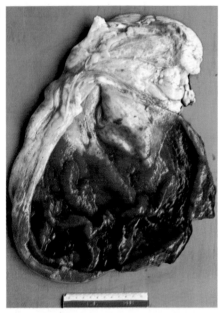

**718 Haemorrhagic cystitis –
urinary bladder: cattle** The urinary
bladder, which contained a reddish
urine, had markedly thickened walls
due to congestion and haemorrhage
in the mucosa.

Differential diagnosis: Chronic
vesicular haematuria.

Decision: Approval with elimination
of the urinary bladder.

719

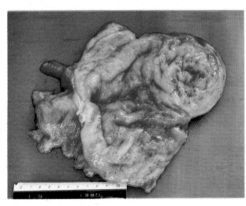

**719 Chronic cystitis –
urinary bladder: cattle** The
bladder's mucosa was pleated
and the whole wall thickened,
rigid and difficult to distend.
These lesions were indicative
of a chronic inflammation
which, the haemorrhages
suggested, were undergoing
periodic activation.

Decision: Approval with
elimination of the urinary
bladder.

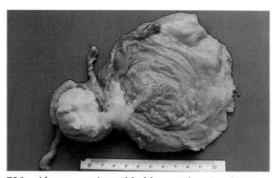

720 Abscess – urinary bladder: cattle An abscess 3 cm in diameter was identified at the point where the ureters terminate. The wall of the bladder was adapted to the abscess, which assumed a pediculated globular appearance. Inside, it contained a more or less solidified yellowish-green pus.

Bacteriological examination of the pus: This showed *Escherichia coli*.

Decision: Approval with elimination of the urinary bladder, because no other lesions or changes were present.

1 Leiomyoma – urinary bladder: tle The opening of the bladder ealed a globular light pink plasia which was fixed in the ll, assuming the characteristics of ign tumours of the smooth scle.

cision: Approval with elimination he urinary bladder.

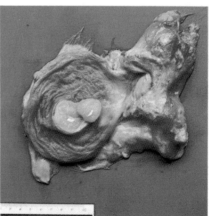

722

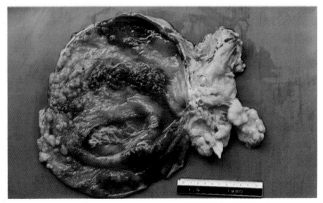

722 Chronic haematuria (malignant evolution) – urinary bladder: cattle The opening of this thick-walled bladder of haemorrhagic content revealed multiple polypoid nodules in the mucosa, haemorrhagic in some areas. Haemorrhagic ulcers could also be seen resulting from necrosis of the mucosa.

Differential diagnosis: Haemorrhagic cystitis; Polypoid cystitis.

Decision: Total condemnation.

723

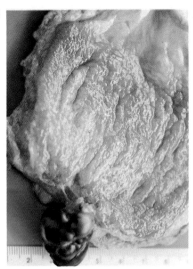

723 Melanotic carcinoma – urinary bladder: cattle In the external wall of the bladder, an ovoid black and shiny neoplasm 3 cm in diameter was identified with characteristics of the melanotic neoplasia.

Differential diagnosis: Haematoma.

Decision: Total condemnation.

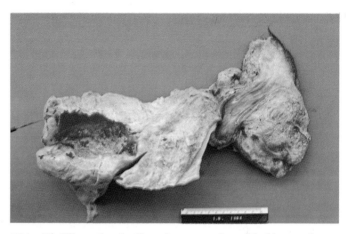

724   Undifferentiated cell carcinoma – urinary bladder: cattle
The bladder, whose walls were thickened and the surface
granular, showed an irregular haemorrhagic mucosa, due to the
development of a carcinoma.

Decision: Total condemnation.

9: The genitalia

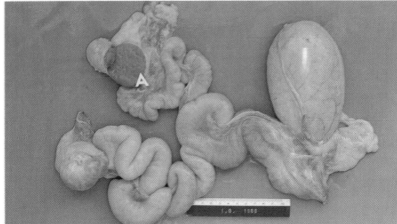

725   Hermaphroditism – genital apparatus: sow   Post-mortem examination revealed that the genital apparatus, particularly the uterus and vagina, was atresic. In the area of insertion of the ovaries, two globular masses were seen with the appearance of testicles. Their incision confirmed that the internal structure was similar to normal testicles, but slightly more reddish.

Differential diagnosis: Ovarian neoplasia; Ovaritis.

Decision: Approval with elimination of the genital apparatus.

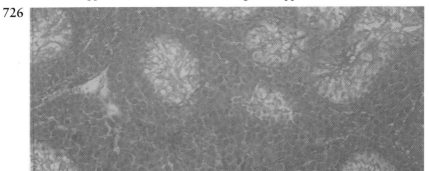

726   Hermaphroditism – intra-abdominal testicle: sow   The seminiferous tubules are reduced to their wall of connective tissue. No Sertoli cells or germinative epithelium were found. On the other hand, the interstitial Leydig cells were very abundant, completely surrounding the seminiferous tubules. H. & E.

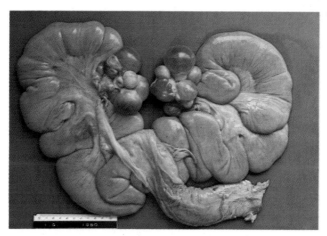

727 Ovarian cysts and dilatation of the uterus – ovary and uterus: sow The wall of the uterus was atonic resulting in the increase in calibre. Both ovaries had cysts.

Differential diagnosis: Cystadenoma.

Decision: Approval with elimination of the genital organs.

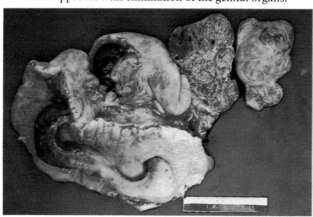

728 Ovaritis – ovary and uterus: cow The ovary was enlarged and the uterine walls distended. The ovary had an excessively large yellow body, whose section showed inflammatory lesions. The opening of the uterus revealed a gelatinous matter, with yellowish as well as dark brown areas, surrounding a foreign body which extended from one horn to the other.

Differential diagnosis: Ovarian neoplasia (in the ovary).

Decision: Approval with elimination of the uterus and ovary.

729

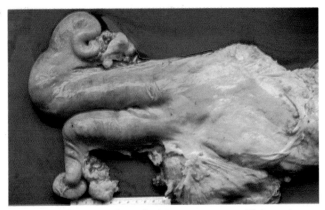

729   Pearl disease (tuberculosis) – ovary: cow   Tuberculous nodules were fixed in the serosa of the uterus. Identical nodules were seen at the surface of the left ovary. All serosae were involved in the process.

Differential diagnosis: Mesothelioma; Actinobacillosis; Parasitic granulomas.

Decision: Total condemnation.

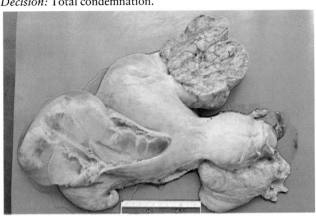

730   Granulosa cell tumour – ovary: cow   This was a gravid uterus in the third month of pregnancy. The right ovary showed a granulosa cell tumour, which deeply modified its normal structure making it appear as an orangy solid firm mass.

Decision: Total condemnation.

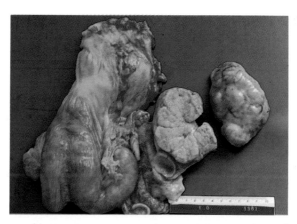

731   Granulosa cell tumour – ovary: cow   The bosselated neoplasia was surrounded by a delicate fibrous capsule, through which the tumour's vasculature was clearly noticed. The cut surface was yellowish-orange and the tissue arranged in nodules separated by connective tissue.

Differential diagnosis: Ovaritis.

Decision: Total condemnation.

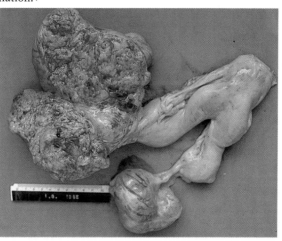

732   Granulosa cell tumour – ovary: mule   Contrasting with the volume of the uterus, always small in these hybrids, two ovaries can be seen, much enlarged due to the development of granulosa cell tumours.

Differential diagnosis: Ovaritis.

Decision: Total condemnation.

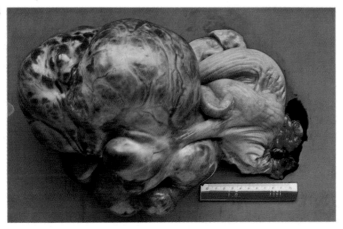

733 Ovarian neoplasia – ovary: cow Attached to a normal uterus a very large grey-red mass was identified. As it showed fluctuation it was thought to be an ovarian cyst.

Hypothetical diagnosis: Ovarian cyst; Granulosa cell tumour; Cystadenoma.

 734

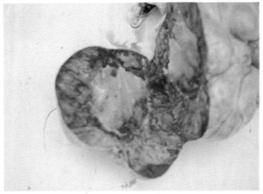

734 Granulosa cell tumour – ovary: cow The incision of the large mass shown in 733 revealed the presence of a large amount of fluid and a solid structure whose central area was bright-yellow and gelatinous, surrounded by a neoplastic-like firm brownish tissue.

Decision: Total condemnation.

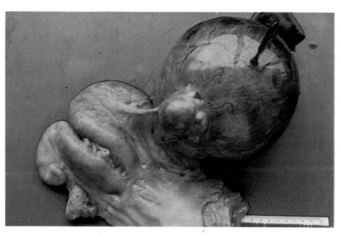

735   Adenocarcinoma – ovary: cow   A voluminous cystic formation developed from the ovary, whose fluctuation seemed to be an ovarian cyst. Incision produced a bloody fluid and showed that the wall of the neoplasia, which appeared to be a fibrous capsule, was surrounding limited areas of lardaceous dark-red tissue.

Differential diagnosis: Ovarian cyst.

Decision: Total condemnation.

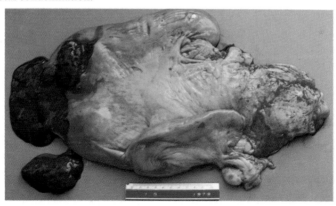

736   Post-partum involution – uterus: cow   The uterus was dilated, with flaccid walls, a bloody content and a few cotyledons in involution.

Differential diagnosis: Haematosalpinx.

Decision: Approval with elimination of the uterus.

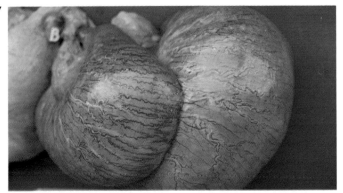

737 Physometra – uterus: cow The uterine walls, which were distended by a large amount of gas under pressure, showed, after incision, a serous-haemorrhagic infiltration of the submucosa. The gaseous distention also involved the peritoneum, where a few gas-containing cysts were identified. B: ovary. Detection of antibiotics in the kidney and carcase was positive.

Decision: Total condemnation.

If the detection of antibiotics had been negative it would have been necessary to determine the bacterial contamination of the carcase and viscera, in order to reach a proper decision.

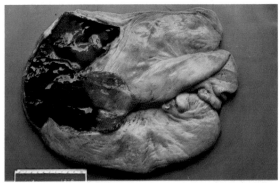

738 Haematosalpinx metrorrhagia – uterus: cow The dilated uterus, with clear atony of its walls, showed after incision a considerable amount of coagulated blood which extended towards the oviduct.

Differential diagnosis: Endometritis; Post-partum involution.

Decision: Approval with elimination of the uterus.

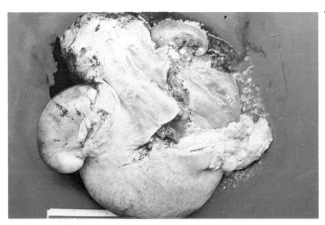

739   Retained placenta – uterus: cow   The uterine horns were markedly swollen and the incision revealed a yellowish-white transparent fluid, odourless, with numerous yellow fibrin-like fragments of placenta in suspension. No signs of inflammation were present.

Differential diagnosis: Endometritis.

Decision: Approval with elimination of the uterus.

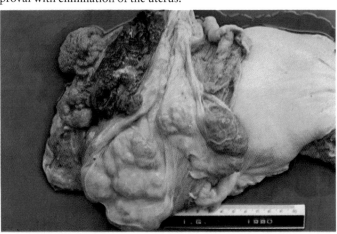

740   Retained placenta – uterus: cow   The opening of the uterus showed parts of fetal sacs, whose caruncles were still attached to the cotyledons (placentomas), although in some areas they had already been detached. Recent birth. No signs of inflammation were present.

Decision: Approval with elimination of the uterus.

741

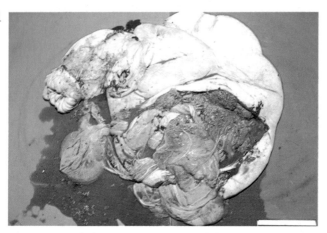

741 Retained placenta – uterus: cow The uterus was dilated with flaccid whitish walls. The incision showed fetal membranes and brownish cotyledons in a considerable amount of altered bloody liquid, which exhaled a fetid smell. The iliac lymph nodes showed signs of reaction.

Decision: Total condemnation.

742

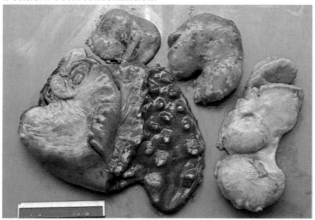

742 Acute metritis – uterus: cow The uterine mucosa was congested. The raised nodules, which corresponded to the final stage of involution of the cotyledons, had a small central yellowish-white purulent focus. Lymphadenitis occurred simultaneously in the iliac and lumbar lymph nodes.

Differential diagnosis: Brucellosis.

Decision: Total condemnation.

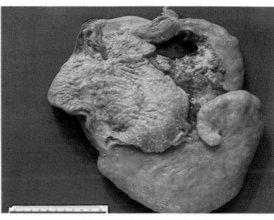

743 Purulent metritis – uterus: cow The uterus was dilated with atonic and delicate walls. The opening showed an oedematous mucosa, pinkish-grey, covered by a greenish-yellow pus. Lymphadenitis occurred simultaneously in the iliac lymph nodes.

Differential diagnosis: Pyometra.

Decision: Total condemnation.

744

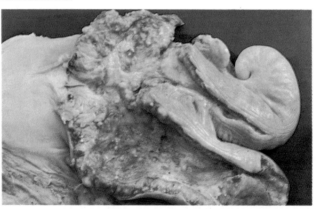

744 Tuberculous metritis (chronic evolution) – uterus: cow The opening of this hypertrophic uterus, whose walls were thickened, showed the mucosa partially covered with a mucopurulent matter, identical to caseum, under which numerous nodules were noticed. Caseous material was identified within the uterine wall, and deeper down, included in fibrous tissue, numerous tubercles were found.

Decision: Approval with elimination of the organ.

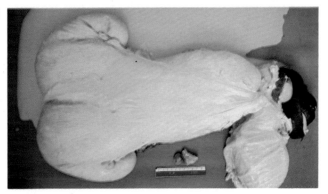

745 Pyometra – uterus: cow The uterine walls, particularly in the body, were distended due to the accumulation of large quantities of a liquid odourless, yellow pus, which drained after the incision. The iliac lymph nodes did not present signs of inflammation.
Bacteriological examination of the pus and the regional lymph nodes in aerobiosis and anaerobiosis: This was negative.

Differential diagnosis: Purulent endometritis.

Decision: Approval with elimination of the uterus.

746

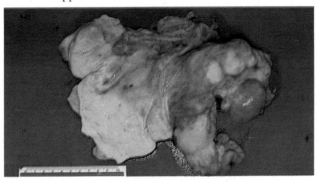

746 Leiomyoma – uterus: sow The uterus showed irregularly thickened pearly-white walls of neoplastic appearance. A brownish firm ovoid mass was identified over the left ovary.

Differential diagnosis: Neoplasia; Metritis.

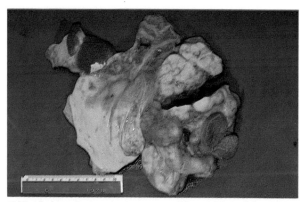

747 Leiomyoma – uterus: sow The section of the thickened horns of **746** showed an area of smooth cut surface, pearly-white and shiny, which corresponded to a leiomyoma. The ovoid mass was an atrophic testicle. The animal was hermaphrodite.

Decision: Approval with elimination of the uterus.

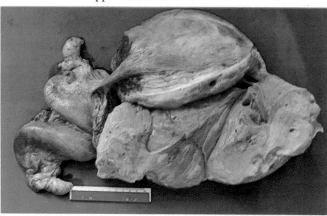

748 Fibromyoma – uterus: cow A mass surrounded by a fibrous capsule, was located inside the uterus. Its consistency was relatively soft, elastic and the section showed a not very compact tissue, the colour varying from yellow to salmon-pink.

Decision: Approval with elimination of the uterus.

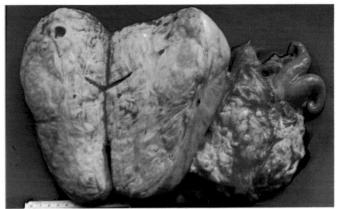

749   Leiomyoma – urogenital organs: ewe   A very firm encapsulated neoplasia was identified in the pelvic cavity attached to the urinary bladder. It had a white cut surface, with fasciculated architecture, typical of leiomyomas.

Decision: Approval with elimination of the uterus and urinary bladder.

750

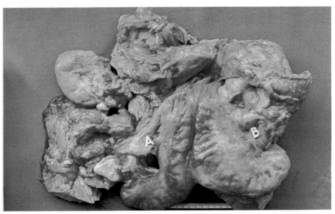

750   Undifferentiated cell carcinoma – uterus: cow   The walls of this uterus were considerably hypertrophic and contained small yellow masses, similar to fat tissue. The histopathological diagnosis was of an undifferentiated cell carcinoma. A and B: ovaries.

Differential diagnosis: Metritis.

Decision: Total condemnation.

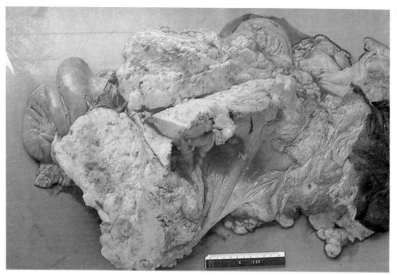

751 Adenocarcinoma – cervix: cow A large pale-yellow tumour, with firm consistency, developed from the cervix. Metastases were present in numerous organs.

Decision: Total condemnation.

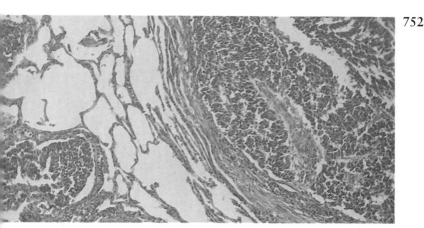

752 Metastasis of an adenocarcinoma of the cervix and lung: cow The pulmonary parenchyma was in some areas compressed by the high development of the metastasis of an adenocarcinoma of the uterus. H. & E.

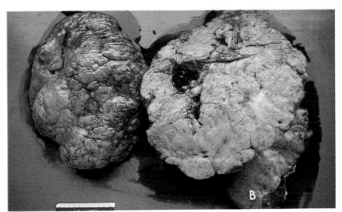

753 Undifferentiated cell sarcoma – uterus: cow This was a very large neoplasia, whose section showed it to be made up of yellow tissue with a few outstanding milky-white small areas of connective tissue. The section of a uterine horn can be seen eccentrically placed in the cut surface. B: uterus.

Differential diagnosis: Granulosa cell tumour; Benign connective tissue tumour

Decision: Total condemnation.

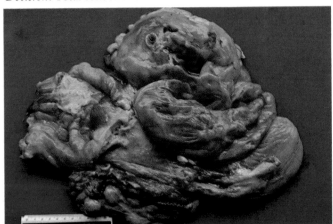

754 Leiomyosarcoma – uterus: cow The uterus was hypertrophic due to the increase in thickness of its walls, which were very firm and pinkish-yellow, suggesting the existence of a neoplasia. Section of the organ revealed a smooth shiny mucosa. This cow had recently aborted, as can be inferred by the presence of fetal sacs and cotyledons.

Differential diagnosis: Metritis.

Decision: Total condemnation.

402

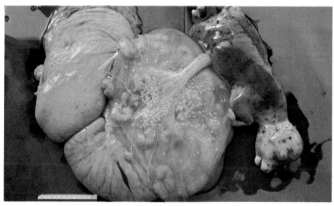

755 Fetal hydrops – uterus: cow The incision of this pregnant uterus plus fetal membranes uncovered a fetus with marked anasarca and subcutaneous haemorrhages. In the amnion, particularly near the umbilical cord, large numbers of small white masses were identified. They corresponded to deposits of keratin which are considered normal.

Differential diagnosis: Brucellosis.

Decision: Approval with elimination of the uterus and its content.
Note: The maternal internal iliac lymph nodes were not reactive.

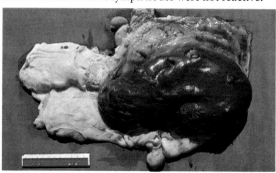

756 Fetal mummification – uterus: cow The uterus was occupied by a mummified fetus with an identifiable head, trunk and outline of limbs. The remains of the fetus showed a sticky soft consistency.

Decision: Approval with elimination of the uterus and its content.

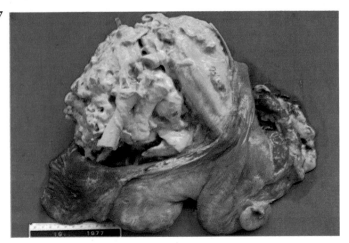

757 Fetal maceration – uterus: cow The uterus was filled with fetal bones mixed with greenish-grey purulent matter. The wall of the uterus, which was perfectly adapted to its content, was affected by a congestive inflammatory reaction. The regional lymph nodes presented acute lymphadenitis.

Decision: Total condemnation.

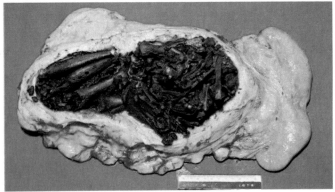

758 Advanced fetal maceration – uterus: cow The uterus was filled with an agglomerate of a fetus's bones, whose soft tissues were totally reabsorbed. No signs of inflammation were present.

Decision: Approval with elimination of the uterus and its content.

759   Cyst – vagina: cow   The longitudinal section of the vagina uncovered a small ovoid structure, arising from the mucosa, that showed fluctuation. The incision showed it was a thin-walled cyst of non-purulent greyish content, liquid and odourless.

Decision: Approval with elimination of the vagina.

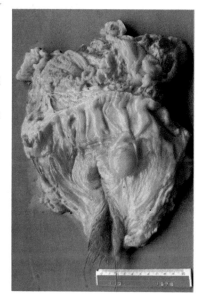

760   Fibroleiomyosarcoma – vagina: cow   A large neoplasia was formed from the wall of the vagina, yellow, dull, of poorly defined limits and firm consistency.

Decision: Total condemnation.

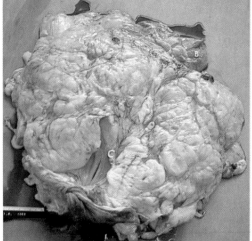

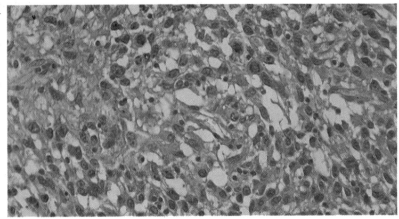

761 Fibroleiomyosarcoma – vagina: cow This neoplasia of the uterine wall is microscopically characterized by a marked histological malignancy, with frequent mitosis and a few abnormally large cells. H. & E.

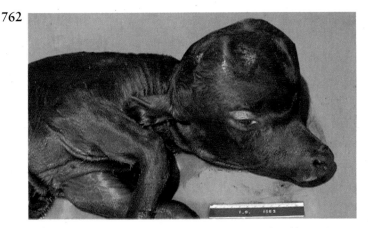

762 Hydrocephalus – bovine: fetus Congenital malformation leading to swelling of the skull due to marked changes in the development of the brain and abnormal accumulation of fluid.

Decision: Approval of the maternal carcase, head and viscera and elimination of the fetus.

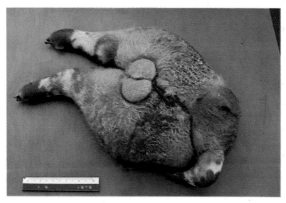

763 Fetal malformation – ovine: fetus This malformation of the *Acephalus* family, genus *Peracephalus*, was removed from the uterus of a ewe.

Decision: Approval of the maternal carcase, head and viscera with elimination of the malformation.

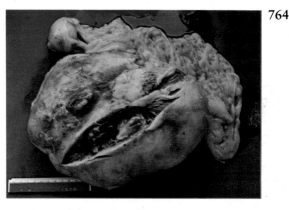

764 Intra-abdominal neoformation: sow A large ovoid mass was located in the abdominal cavity, attached to the omentum. It had a fibrous capsule and contained solidified material.

Differential diagnosis: Cyst; Neoplasia; Lymphadenitis.

765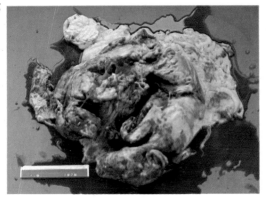

765 Encysted fetus: sow The opening of the mass presented in **764** showed that it contained two fetuses. The absence of fetal membranes and the advanced stage of development of the fetuses suggested a rupture of the uterus and consequent passage of the fetuses to the abdominal cavity, where an inflammatory reaction built up around them.

Decision: Approval with elimination of the fetuses.

766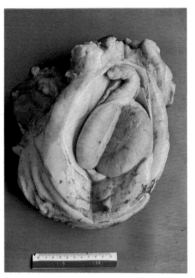

766 Fibrinous periorchitis – scrotum: b A considerable amount of yellow fibrinou exudate accumulated around the testicles an exudative inflammatory reaction involving the testicular tunicae.

Decision: Approval with elimination of t testicles.

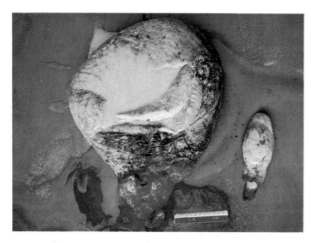

767 Abscess – scrotum: sheep The scrotum was markedly distended and showed some fluctuation. The incision revealed an accumulation of a yellowish fluid pus, surrounded by a highly fibrous pyogenic membrane. The regional lymph nodes were reactive.
Bacteriological examination of the pus: This showed *Escherichia coli* and *Clostridium perfringens*.

Decision: Total condemnation.

768 Roeckl's granuloma – scrotum: bull
The incision of a swollen scrotum revealed a purulent inflammatory reaction that developed from the tail of the epididymis. The reaction was extensive to the tunicae which showed lesions of various ages, from congestion to fibrosis, depending on their distance from the original inflammatory focus.

Differential diagnosis: Spermatocele; Tuberculosis.

Decision: Approval if no other lesions are present, with elimination of the testicles.

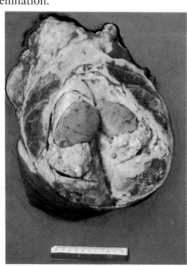

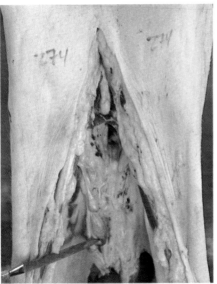

769 Cryptorchidism – testicle (carcase): swine In the abdominal cavity of a swine, a testicle was found, which was atrophic; this is common in cases of cryptorchidism. The meat did not give off a sexual odour.

Decision: Approval with elimination of the testicle.

The removal of samples for frying, roasting and boiling tests should be done from the fat, muscles of the thigh, intercostal muscles with covering fat and perirenal fat. The roasting test can be performed on the carcase itself with an instrument similar to a soldering iron.

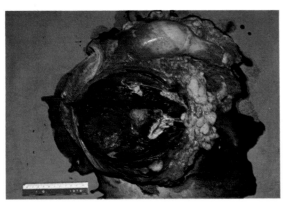

770 Haematocele – testicle: bull A testicle suffered a severe traumatic injury, causing a considerable haematocele.

Decision: Approval with elimination of the testicle.

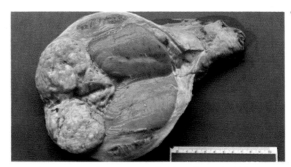

771   Spermatocele – testicle: bull   The tail of the epididymis was thickened and its section showed numerous whitish nodules which contained a yellowish caseous-like material.

Differential diagnosis: Tuberculosis of the epididymis; Roeckl's granuloma.

Decision: Approval with elimination of the testicles.

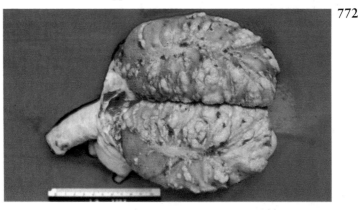

772   Roeckl's granuloma – testicle: bull   The incision of this swollen testicle showed a large number of bulging necrotic foci with dystrophic calcification. These lesions were similar to calcified caseous tuberculosis both macroscopically and microscopically, but it was not possible to identify acid-fast bacilli.

Differential diagnosis: Tuberculosis; Spermatocele; Orchitis in brucellosis.

Decision: Approval, if no other lesions are present, with elimination of the testicles.
A careful observation of the muscles should be made to search for lesions of nodular necrosis.

773

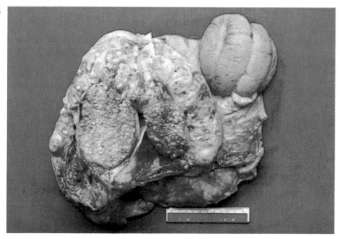

774

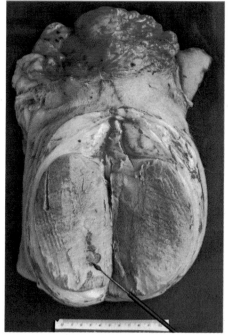

773 Purulent orchitis – testicle: bull The incision of the testicles showed a unilateral purulent infection involving the tunicae, which also displayed marked fibrosis. The regional lymph nodes showed signs of reaction.

Decision: Total condemnation or, alternatively, approval after heat treatment, subject to the results of the laboratory examination, with elimination of the testicles.

774 Necrotizing orchitis – testicle: bull One of the testicles was markedly hypertrophic due to a necrotic inflammation. The incision showed a congested parenchyma with small foci of softened tissue. The regional lymph nodes were slightly swollen.

Decision: Approval subject to the results of the laboratory examination (brucellosis), with elimination of the testicles.

775 Necropurulent orchitis – testicle: bull The testicle was reduced to small reddish-yellow foci contained in a cavity with very thick fibrous walls. The regional lymph nodes were reactive.

Differential diagnosis: Orchitis in brucellosis; Tuberculous orchitis.

Bacteriological examination of the testicle fragments: This was *Staphylococcus* coagulase positive.

Decision: Total condemnation.

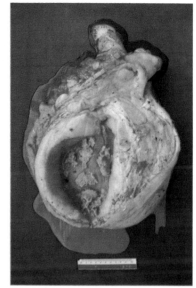

775

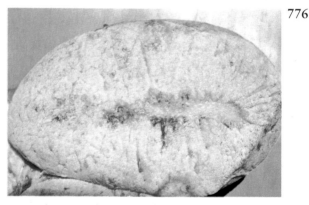

776

776 Chronic orchitis – testicle: bull This testicle of normal volume and firm consistency, presented a yellow cut surface where the normal tubular structure was clearly seen together with a considerable increase in connective tissue. These lesions corresponded to tubular necrosis with fibrosis of the interstitial tissue.

Decision: Approval with elimination of the testicles.

413

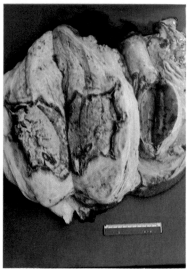

777   **Orchitis – brucellosis – testicles: b**
Palpation of the scrotum revealed a firm
swollen testicle. The incision showed tha
the parenchyma had been replaced by
yellow necrotic matter, surrounded by
fibrous tissue. No reaction was seen in th
regional lymph nodes.

Differential diagnosis: Tuberculous
orchitis.

Decision: Approval with elimination of t
testicles and regional lymph nodes.
When *Brucella melitensis* is isolated and
regional lymphadenitis is present, the bes
decision is total condemnation. Approva
may be considered with thermal treatmer
and elimination of the testicles and regio
lymph nodes. Professional risk should al
be considered.

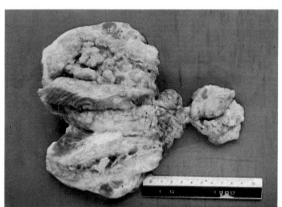

778   **Chronic tuberculosis – testicles: bull**   The
longitudinal section of one testicle uncovered calcified
caseous lesions of tuberculosis together with a marked
fibrous reaction of the parenchyma, which is almost
completely destroyed.

Differential diagnosis: Orchitis in brucellosis;
Nonspecific orchitis.

Decision: Approval with elimination of the testicles.

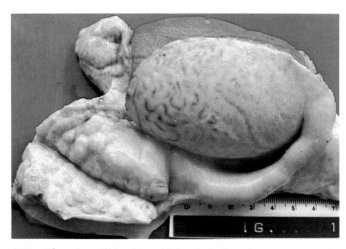

779   Chronic epididymitis epididymis: bull   The incision of
the tail of this hypertrophic epididymis showed a clear increase in
connective tissue around the ductus epididymis, which protruded
above the cut surface.

Differential diagnosis: Tuberculosis; Spermatocele.

Decision: Approval with elimination of the testicles.

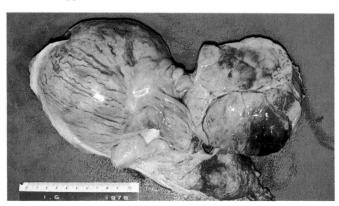

780   Malignant seminoma – testicle: horse   There is a
bosselated structure under the tunica albuginea. The incision
showed a yellowish shiny tissue, with multiple haemorrhagic foci.

Differential diagnosis: Acute orchitis.

Decision: Total condemnation.

781

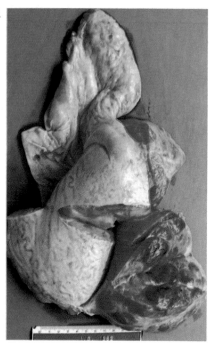

781 Malignant seminoma – testicles: bull The incision of this extremely swollen testicle showed a moderately congested parenchyma with small reddish-brown well individualized, firm shiny nodules.

Differential diagnosis: Orchitis.

Decision: Total condemnation.

782

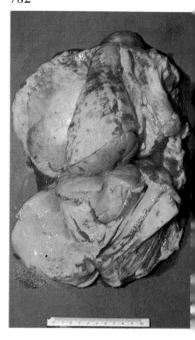

782 Undifferentiated cell sarcoma – testicle: bull This hypertrophic testicle was affected by an extensive fibrinous inflammation of the tunicae. Small pinkish raised areas were noticed at the surface of the tunica albuginea. Their limits were well-defined and they had a tumorous appearance, penetrating in some zones into the testicle itself. Similar lesions were found in the walls of the scrotum and in between the fibrinous exudate.

Decision: Total condemnation.

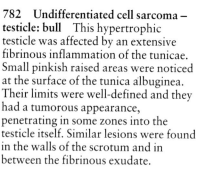

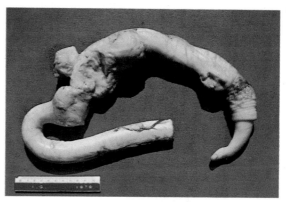

783 Multiple abscesses – penis: bull Alongside the penis were several swellings containing greenish-yellow pus. The regional lymph nodes were not reactive.

Bacteriology of the pus: Proteus vulgaris and *Pseudomonas sp.*

Decision: Approval with elimination of the penis.

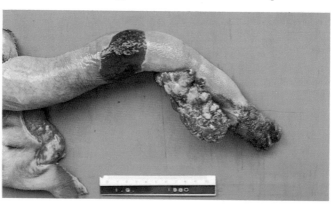

784 Fibroepithelioma – penis: ox Near the apex of the penis, which showed necrotic lesions, a papilloma-like mass was found, the colour of which varied from dark-pink to pearly white. A congested ulcer was noticed in the middle of the organ, which histopathological examination revealed to be tumorous.

Differential diagnosis: Papilloma.

Decision: Total condemnation.

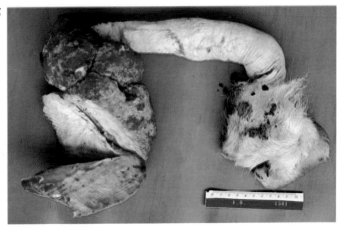

785 Fibrosarcoma – penis: ox A large globular mass formed in the glans of the penis. Its surface was irregularly granular, with haemorrhages and necrotic foci. The incision showed a whitish fibrous and homogenous cut surface.

Differential diagnosis: Papilloma.

Decision: Total condemnation.

10: The nervous system

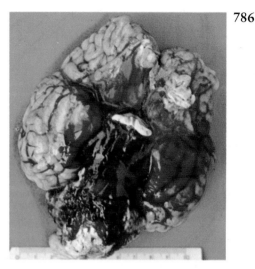

786 Subdural haemorrhages* – brain: cattle Brain of an animal which was admitted for emergency slaughter in a comatose condition, showing extensive subdural haemorrhages.

Hypothetical diagnosis: Listeriosis; Viral encephalitis; Post-vaccinal reaction; Lead poisoning; Cranial traumatism.

Decision: The animal was condemned at the ante-mortem inspection.

*Similar lesions were identified in other animals from the same farm.

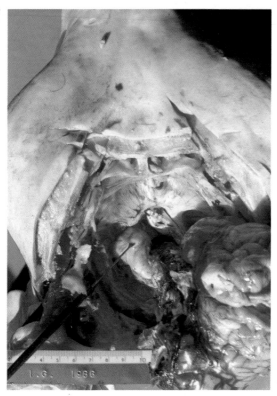

787 Abscess – brain: calf The opening of the skull revealed the existence of a pouch at the base of the brain, to which it was adherent near the hypophyseal fossa of the sphenoid bone. It was made up of fibrous tissue the palpation of which revealed some fluctuation. The incision showed it contained a fluid yellowish pus.

Decision: Approval with elimination of the brain.

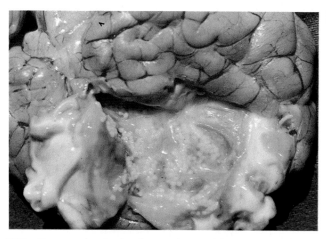

788 Cόenurosis – brain: sheep A parasitic cyst was located in the brain, causing the nervous symptoms which were observed in the ante-mortem inspection. The cyst contained a transparent fluid and numerous white scolices.

Decision: Approval with elimination of the head.

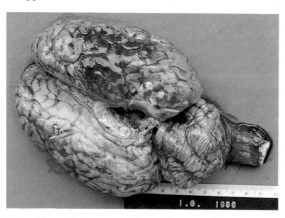

789 Choroid plexus papilloma: horse The dissection of the brain was carried out because the animal presented nervous symptoms in the ante-mortem inspection. A neoplasia of the choroid plexuses was noticed, at the III and IV ventricles.

Differential diagnosis: Haematoma.

Decision: Approval with elimination of the brain.

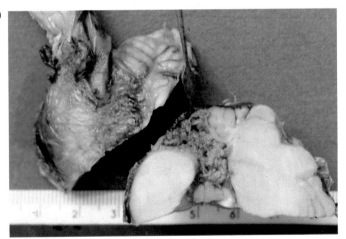

790 Choroid plexus papilloma: horse When sectioning the brain shown in the previous picture, after a few days fixation in 10% formalin, the neoplasia located in the IV ventricle, could be seen in greater detail.

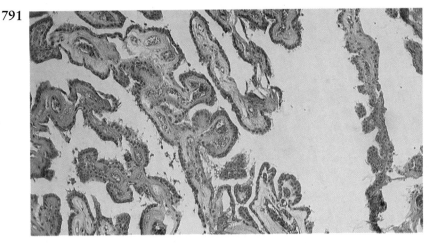

791 Choroid plexus papilloma: horse A benign tumour formed from the choroid plexuses, which due to its morphological characteristics, was classified as a papilloma. H.&E.

**792   Malignant melanosis –
meninges: cattle**   At the lumbar-
sacral region the meninges were
highly infiltrated with melanin in a
case of malignant melanosis.

Decision: Total condemnation.

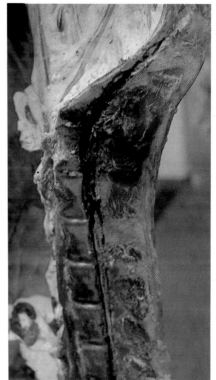

**793   Malignant melanosis –
meninges: cattle**   The pia mater
was infiltrated with melanin, which
was also visible in the brain fissures.
H.&E.

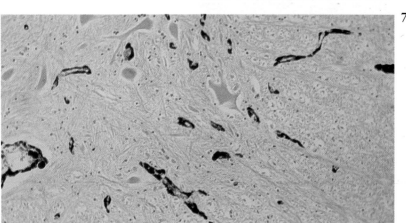

794

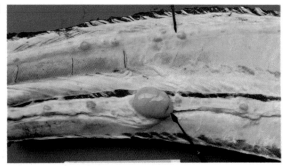

794 Neurofibromatosis – nerves: ribs: cattle Several fusiform masses developed from the intercostal nerves, most of them 5 cm long and 3 cm wide, which corresponded to nodules of neurofibromatosis.

Differential diagnosis: Metastasis of malignant neoplasia; Cysts; Acute miliary tuberculosis; Cysticercosis.

Decision: Approval with elimination of the lesions.

795

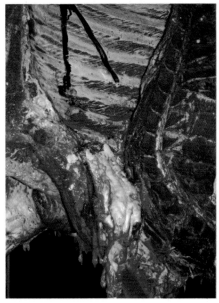

795 Neurofibromatosis – nerve – carcase: cattle The presence of a small hyalin nodule which was attached to an intercostal nerve, suggested the removal of the brachi plexus. This was accomplished by severing the insertion of the scalenu muscles in the first rib, and pulling the brachial plexus, taking off the bridles to neighbouring tissues. This uncommon technique, which avoids the partial disarticulation of the thoracic limb, does not deprecia the carcase. In this case the plexus was transformed into a fusiform mass with tumorous appearance. Extensive lesions of neurofibromatos were also found in the viscera.

Decision: Total condemnation considering the generalization and exuberance of the lesions in the carcase and viscera.

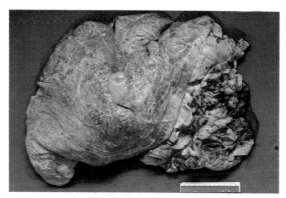

**796 Neurofibromatosis – pneumogastric nerve:
cattle** A large neoplasia, which originated from the
pneumogastric nerve, was found in the mediastinum,
showing continuity with the cranial pulmonary lobes.
Its lardaceous appearance suggested a malignant
tumour but this was not confirmed by the
histopathological examination.

Decision: Approval with elimination of the lungs.

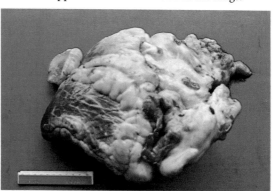

797 Neurofibromatosis – nerves – heart: cattle
Several lesions of neurofibromatosis were found in the
heart shown. An irregular white and firm fusiform
lesion of the aortic plexus can be seen on the right,
deforming the auricle. In the ventricular wall, amongst
the thickened nerves of the cardiac plexus equally
involved, a small fusiform mass can be seen. Finally, on
the left, a nodule of typical internal structure, revealed
by the incision.

Decision: Approval with elimination of the heart and
lungs.

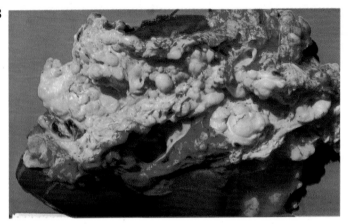

798 Neurofibromatosis – nerve – liver: cattle The caudal
face of the liver was deeply modified by a whitish mass of fibrous
tissue, which included several round or ovoid shiny white nodules
as a consequence of the neoplastic proliferation of the connective
tissue of the neural sheaths.

Decision: Approval, if no other lesions are present, with
elimination of the liver.

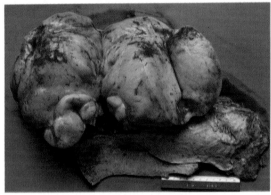

799 Neurofibroma – nerve – spleen: cattle A
spherical tumour, the size of a human head, was
attached to the spleen. The cut surface was yellowish,
smooth and shiny.

Differential diagnosis: Lipoma.

Decision: Approval, if no other lesions are present, with
elimination of the spleen.

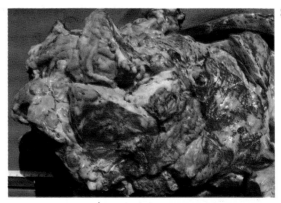

800 Neurofibromatosis – nerve – pancreas: cattle
The pancreas was markedly hypertrophic with several
bosselated areas at the surface. The incision revealed the
presence of a few cords with fusiform pearly and firm
dilatations which are characteristic of
neurofibromatosis.

Decision: Approval with elimination of the pancreas.

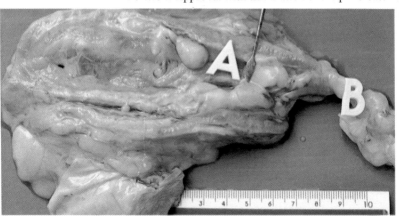

801 Neurofibromatosis – mediastinal lymph node: cattle During inspection,
the incision of a mediastinal lymph node revealed small pearly white round
formations of firm consistency. These were small lesions of neurofibromatosis.

Decision: Approval with elimination of the affected tissues.

802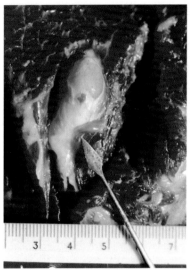

802 Neurofibromatosis – nerve, muscle: cattle Within a muscle of a carcase with disseminated neurofibromatosis, an ovoid mass was identified. The incision showed it was a neoplasia originating from the neural connective tissue cells.

Decision: Total condemnation.

803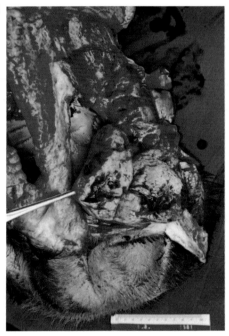

803 Neurofibromatosis – nerve, lower jaw: cattle In the soft tissue of the medial side of the right lower jaw, a globular neoplasia was found. The incision showed it to be made up of a white, shiny tissue of tumorous appearance with a few extensive haemorrhagic foci.

Decision: Approval with elimination of the neoplasia.

04 Neurofibromatosis – nerve, pharynx:
attle A very large encapsulated neoplasia of
ell-defined limits was found in the
haryngeal area. The incision showed it was
ade-up of a white, shiny, tumorous tissue.

ecision: Approval with elimination of the
eoplasia.

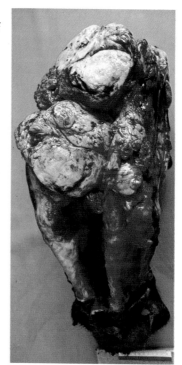

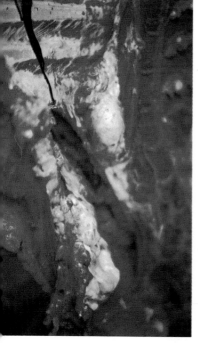

805 Neurofibromatosis – sympathetic
nerve: cattle Underneath the body of
the first dorsal vertebra, a globular
tumour of the sympathetic nerve was
found. The incision showed a lardaceous
homogeneous tissue, typical of the
nuerofibromas. The picture also shows
an area of the brachial plexus with
lesions of neurofibromatosis.

Decision: Approval with elimination of
the affected areas of the nerve.

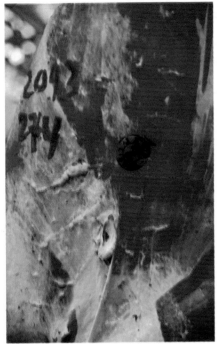

806 Neurofibromatosis – subcutaneous nerves: cattle In the subcutaneous tissue of the costal area, some neural branches were thickened, presenting a few nodules corresponding to lesions of neurofibromatosis. The muscles in the carcase and viscera also presented lesions of neurofibromatosis.

Differential diagnosis: Deep dermatomycosis; Skin sarcomas; Multiple tuberous lymphangiomas.

Decision: Total condemnation.

807 Malignant neurofibromatosis – nerve: cattle Along the pneumogastric nerve at the tracheal level, a large globular swelling was found. The incision showed it had an encephaloid appearance, suggesting malignancy.

Decision: Total condemnation.

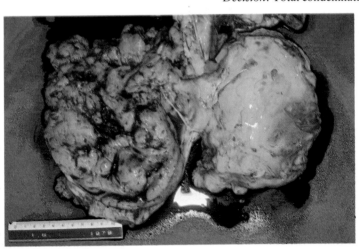

808 Malignant neurofibromatosis plesus aorticus: cattle A large shiny lardaceous tumour, with haemorrhagic foci was located at the base of the heart. It had developed from the plexus aorticus and its macroscopical characteristics were not of a benign neurofibroma.

Decision: Total condemnation.

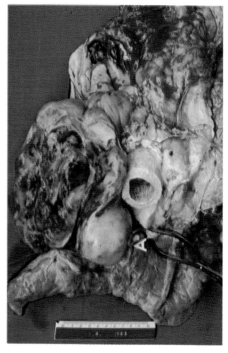

809 Malignant neurofibromatosis – peripheral nerve: cattle Endoneural tumorous growth, characterized by the arrangement of the cells in whorls. H.&E.

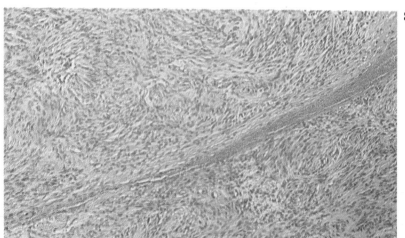

810

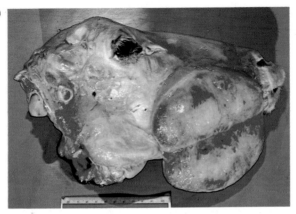

810 Malignant schwannoma – cheek: sheep A globular encapsulated mass was attached to the cheek of a sheep. The incision showed a lardaceous tissue with several small haemorrhages.

Decision: Total condemnation.

811

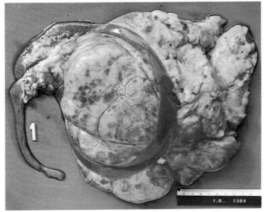

811 Malignant schwannoma – intestine: sheep The histological examination of a voluminous encephaloid mass attached to the small intestine of a sheep, revealed it was a malignant neoplasia of the cells of Schwann.

Differential diagnosis: Lipoma.

Decision: Total condemnation.

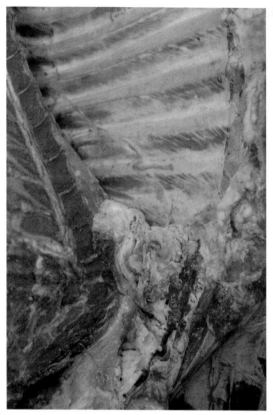

812 Chemoreceptor cell tumour – entrance of the chest: cow At the anterior end of the thorax, in the area of the thymus, a white, shiny, nodular neoplasia was found. A metastasis of the neoplasia was present in the external costal region, behind the scapula.

Differential diagnosis: Neurofibromatosis.

Decision: Total condemnation.

11: The endocrine glands

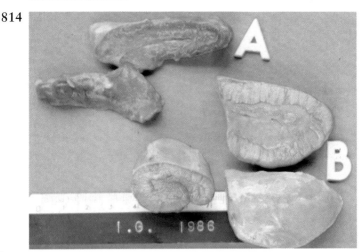

813   Steatosis – adrenal glands: cattle   A – Normal adrenal gland showing clear limits between cortex and medulla.

B – Adrenal gland showing steatosis.
Cortex and medulla were both affected by deposition of fat, showing a uniform yellow colo[ur]. The limits between the two are[as] were not clear. The black pigm[ent] seen in the cortex was melanin.

Differential diagnosis: Amyloidosis.

Decision: Approval, if no othe[r] lesions are present, with elimination of the affected adr[enal] glands.

814   Amyloidosis adrenal glands: cattle   The enlargement of the 'B' adrenal gland was due to hyperplasia of the cortex, the yellow orange colour of which favours the existence of amyloidosis. In 'A', sections of normal adrenal gland can be seen. Similar lesions affected the kidney.

Differential diagnosis: Lipid deposition; Secondary amyloidosis.

Decision: Total condemnation.

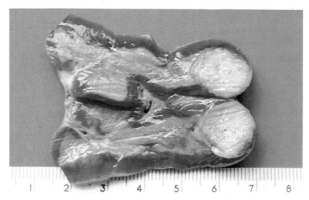

815 Tuberculosis – adrenal gland: cattle A calcified caseous nodule was identified in a pole of this adrenal gland. The lesion destroyed the cortex in the corresponding area, as well as the medulla.

Decision: Approval, if no other lesions are present, with elimination of the adrenal gland.

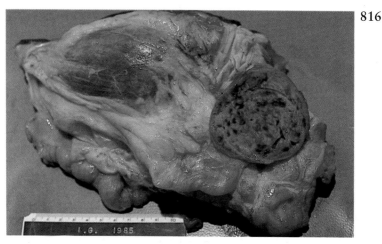

816 Adenoma of the adrenal cortex: horse The organ was hypertrophic and the incision showed a brownish surface with multiple small dark haemorrhages.

Differential diagnosis: Malignant neoplasia.

Decision: Approval with elimination of the adrenal gland.

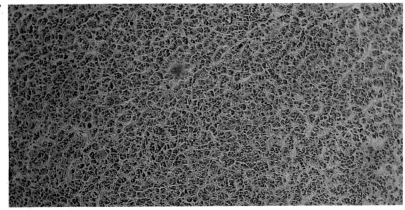

817 Adenoma of the cortex – adrenal glands: horse The highly differentiated cells assume a cord-like disposition, with the morphological characteristics of the cells of the zona fasciculata. H.&E.

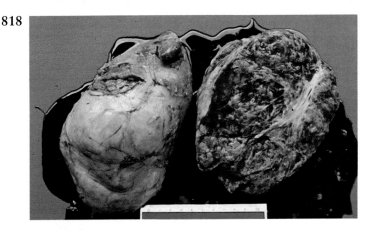

818 Carcinoma of the cortex – adrenal glands: cattle The adrenal gland was extremely hypertrophic, with only one extremity appearing normal, due to the development of a cortical neoplasia. The incision produced a large amount of blood and revealed that the glandular structure was totally destroyed by the proliferation of a tumorous, pink, shiny tissue.

Decision: Total condemnation.

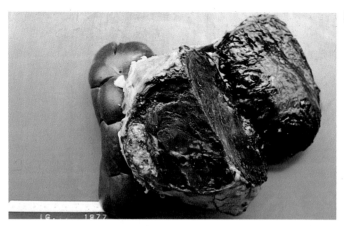

819 Carcinoma of the cortex – adrenal glands: cattle
A large encapsulated globular neoplasia developed from the
cortex of the adrenal gland. Its incision showed it had a
polychromic aspect. Extensive haemorrhages were noticed and
the central area was yellow and gelatinous.

Decision: Total condemnation.

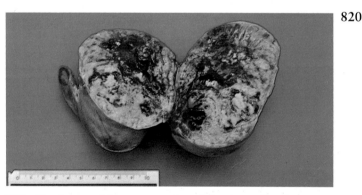

820 Carcinoma of the cortex – adrenal glands: cattle A
cortical neoplasia developed in this adrenal gland leaving only
a small normal portion. Its polychromic aspect is typical and it
was due to the haemorrhages which normally occur in these
tumours. The sulphur-yellow colour present in certain areas of
the tumour is also typical.

Decision: Total condemnation.

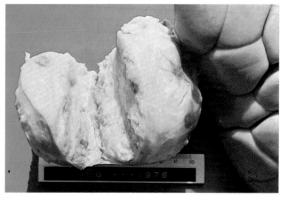

**821 Carcinoma of the cortex – adrenal glands:
cattle** Although infrequently, the cortical carcinoma of
the adrenal gland may assume aspects of uniform
morphology, as in the present case. The neoplasia
presented a fine granular appearance, golden-yellow,
which is justified by the lack of haemorrhages.

Differential diagnosis: Tuberculosis of the renal lymph
node.

Decision: Total condemnation.

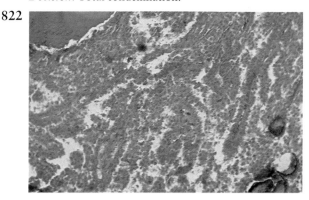

**822 Carcinoma of the cortex – adrenal glands:
cattle** The neoplastic cells were arranged in long
strands, supported by delicate fibrous tissue, a similar
appearance to papillary adenocarcinomas. Small foci of
dystrophic calcification are frequent in these tumours.
H.&E.

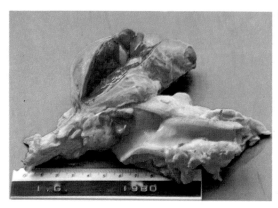

823   Carcinoma of the medulla – adrenal glands: cattle   The adrenal gland was moderately swollen. The incision showed that the medulla was affected by a proliferative lesion with the appearance of a malignant neoplasia. Examination of the neighbouring tissues revealed the infiltrative nature of the neoplasia, which destroyed the wall of the abdominal aorta, penetrating the lumen of the arteria, where it developed, almost obliterating the vessel.

Differential diagnosis: Thrombus in the aorta.

Decision: Total condemnation.

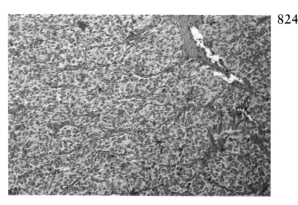

824   Carcinoma of the medulla – adrenal glands: cattle   The cells resulting from the proliferation of the medulla tend to be fusiform with elongated nucleus, arranged in groups separated by a rich capillary rete. H.&E.

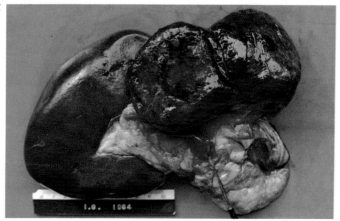

825 Carcinoma of the medulla – adrenal glands: horse Only a small portion of this adrenal gland remained normal (indicated by the probe), the rest of it being affected by a neoplasia of the medulla, the cut surface of which presented several haemorrhages.

Decision: Total condemnation.

826

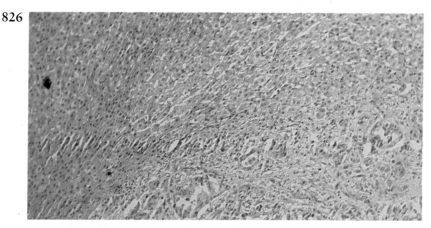

826 Metastasis of adenocarcinoma – adrenal gland: cattle The normal architecture of the adrenal gland was highly disturbed due to the metastatic invasion of an adenocarcinoma of undetermined origin. H.&E.

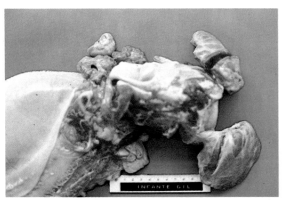

827 Hypertrophy – thyroid: cattle The thyroid glands were considerably swollen. Simultaneously congestive and haemorrhagic lesions were present in the tonsils. Both lesions and others found in the carcase, testicles and adrenal glands were due to the administration of a thyrostatic substance – methylthiouracil.

Differential diagnosis: Thyroid neoplasia; Thyroiditis.

Decision: Total condemnation due to the complete pathological picture and due to the high content of methylthiouracil detected in the carcase.

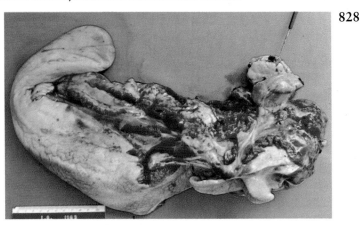

828

828 Parenchymatous goitre – thyroid: horse The histological examination of the thyroid shown in the picture revealed parenchymatous goitre.

Differential diagnosis: Choloid goitre; Neoplasia; Thyroiditis.

Decision: Approval with elimination of the thyroid.

829

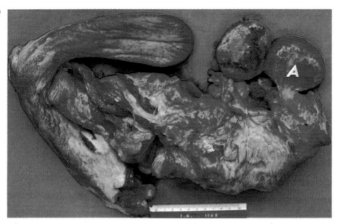

829 Adenoma – thyroid: horse The histological examination of the thyroid shown in the picture revealed a solid follicular adenoma.

Differential diagnosis: Goitre; Thyroiditis.

Decision: Approval with elimination of the thyroid.

830

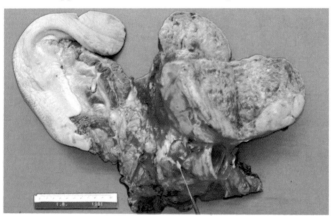

830 Solid follicular carcinoma – thyroid: horse A malignant neoplasia developed in one of the thyroid glands, which was markedly enlarged and encapsulated. The cut surface looked heterogenous, bright yellow just under the capsule. The central area had an appearance of muscle tissue. The probe indicates the normal gland.

Differential diagnosis: Goitre.

Decision: Total condemnation.

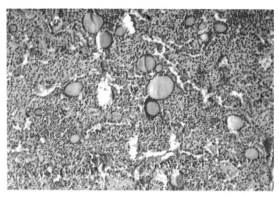

831 Solid follicular carcinoma – thyroid: cattle The
neoplasia presented two distinctive aspects. In the same
area, solid cell cords alternated with follicles, similar to
the ones found in the normal glands. H.&E.

12: The eye

832

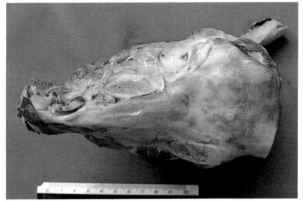

832 Anophthalmos: sheep Congenital disorder.
There is total absence of ocular tissue. There were no
orbital cavities, a slight depression corresponding to
their normal location.

Decision: Approval.

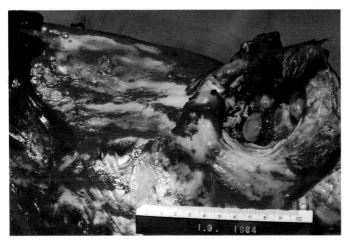

833 Squamous cell carcinoma of the third eyelid – eye: cattle
From the medial canthus of the eye a small neoplasia was formed, lobulated and highly congested with some superficial erosions, secondarily infected.

Differential diagnosis: Bovine infectious keratitis; Unspecific keratitis; Conjunctival rickettsiosis.

Decision: Total condemnation.

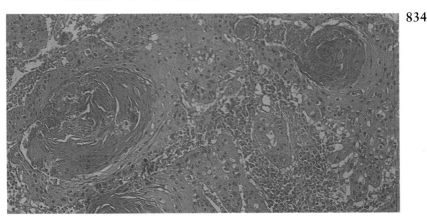

834 Squamous cell carcinoma of the third eyelid – eye: cattle The malpighian epithelium proliferated within a stroma rich in mononucleated lymphoid cells, forming cell cords, which frequently suffered central keratinization in concentric layers. H.&.E.

Appendix: The Bovine Lymphatic System

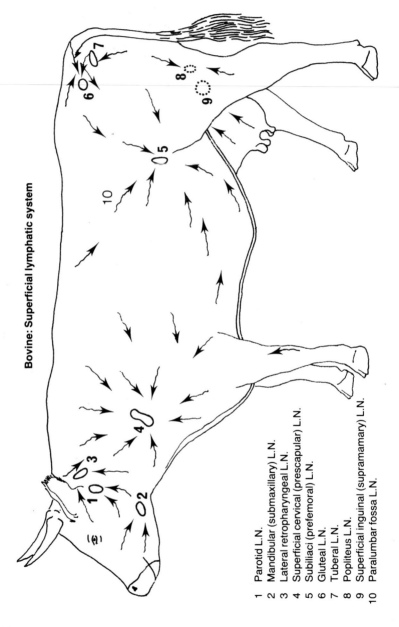

Bovine: Superficial lymphatic system

1 Parotid L.N.
2 Mandibular (submaxillary) L.N.
3 Lateral retropharyngeal L.N.
4 Superficial cervical (prescapular) L.N.
5 Subiliaci (prefemoral) L.N.
6 Gluteal L.N.
7 Tuberal L.N.
8 Popliteus L.N.
9 Superficial inguinal (supramamary) L.N.
10 Paralumbar fossa L.N.

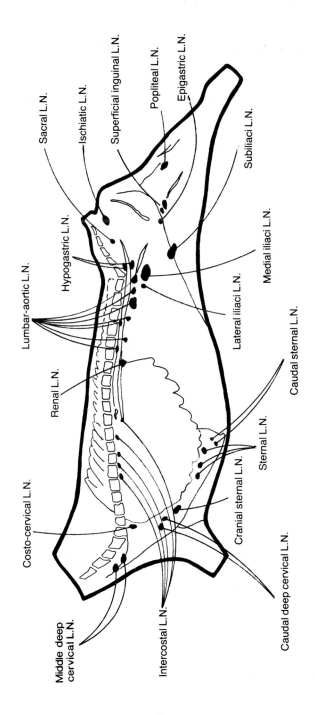

Sacral L.N.

Ischiatic L.N.

Superficial inguinal L.N.

Popliteal L.N.

Epigastric L.N.

Subiliaci L.N.

Hypogastric L.N.

Medial iliaci L.N.

Lumbar-aortic L.N.

Lateral iliaci L.N.

Renal L.N.

Caudal sternal L.N.

Costo-cervical L.N.

Sternal L.N.

Cranial sternal L.N.

Caudal deep cervical L.N.

Middle deep cervical L.N.

Intercostal L.N.

Bovine Half-carcase: superficial lymph nodes

447

INDEX